Christine Huchzermeyer

Energy demands during gamma oscillations in the hippocampus

Christine Huchzermeyer

Energy demands during gamma oscillations in the hippocampus

A study of neuronal activity and mitochondrial function in hippocampal brain slice preparations

Südwestdeutscher Verlag für
Hochschulschriften

Imprint
Any brand names and product names mentioned in this book are subject to trademark, brand or patent protection and are trademarks or registered trademarks of their respective holders. The use of brand names, product names, common names, trade names, product descriptions etc. even without a particular marking in this work is in no way to be construed to mean that such names may be regarded as unrestricted in respect of trademark and brand protection legislation and could thus be used by anyone.

Publisher:
Südwestdeutscher Verlag für Hochschulschriften
is a trademark of
Dodo Books Indian Ocean Ltd., member of the OmniScriptum S.R.L Publishing group
str. A.Russo 15, of. 61, Chisinau-2068, Republic of Moldova Europe
Printed at: see last page
ISBN: 978-3-8381-2051-5

Zugl. / Approved by: Berlin, Charité-Universitätsmedizin Berlin, Diss., 2010

Copyright © Christine Huchzermeyer
Copyright © 2010 Dodo Books Indian Ocean Ltd., member of the OmniScriptum S.R.L Publishing group

Contents

		Page
1	INTRODUCTION	1
1.1	Neuronal activity in the hippocampus	1
1.2	Gamma oscillations	2
1.3	Oxidative energy metabolism in the brain	5
1.4	Monitoring of neuronal activity and mitochondrial redox state	7
2	AIM OF THE STUDY	11
3	MATERIALS AND METHODS	13
3.1	Organotypic hippocampal slice cultures (OHSCs)	13
3.2	Acute hippocampal slices	14
3.3	Solutions and recordings	14
3.4	O_2-sensitive microelectrode	16
3.5	Fluorescence recordings of NAD(P)H and FAD	17
3.6	Fluorescence recordings of rhodamine-123	18
3.7	Chronic rotenone treatment of OHSCs and Fluoro-Jade B staining	18
3.8	Calculations and statistics	20
4	RESULTS	21
4.1	Gamma oscillations in rat OHSCs and acute mouse hippocampal slices induced by acetylcholine	21
4.2	Neuronal activity and its sensitivity to decreases in tissue pO_2	25
4.2.1	Gamma oscillations	25
4.2.2	Spontaneous network activity and evoked local field potential responses	27
4.3	Changes in interstitial pO_2 and mitochondrial redox state	29
4.3.1	Quantification of interstitial pO_2	29
4.3.2	Quantification of NAD(P)H and FAD fluorescence	32
4.4	O_2 consumption and mitochondrial redox state during gamma oscillations	36

4.4.1	Interstitial pO_2 during spontaneous activity and during gamma oscillations in acute mouse hippocampal slices	36
4.4.2	O_2 consumption during gamma oscillations in rat OHSCs	39
4.4.3	O_2 consumption of low Mg^{2+}-induced epileptiform activity	43
4.4.4	Mitochondrial redox state during gamma oscillations	45
4.5	Chronic rotenone model	48
4.5.1	Chronic rotenone application and neuronal cell death	48
4.5.2	Mitochondrial redox responses during chronic rotenone application	49
5	DISCUSSION	52
5.1	Gamma oscillations and their sensitivity to changes in tissue pO_2	53
5.2	O_2 consumption during gamma oscillations	55
5.3	O_2 availability in hippocampal slice preparations	56
5.4	Mitochondrial redox state as a marker for functional performance of mitochondria	58
5.5	Mitochondrial redox state during gamma oscillations	59
5.6	Rotenone-induced alterations in mitochondrial redox state	60
5.7	Functional consequences	62
6	SUMMARY	63
7	ZUSAMMENFASSUNG	65
8	REFERENCES	67
9	ACKNOWLEDGMENTS	77

List of abbrevations

ACh	acetylcholine
ACSF	artificial cerebrospinal fluid
ATP	adenosine triphosphate
CA1, CA2, CA3	cornu ammonis 1, 2, 3
CC	cytochrome c
div	days in vitro
ETC	electron transport chain
FAD	flavin adenine dinucleotide
FJB	Fluoro-Jade B
FWHM	full width at half maximum
GABA	gamma-aminobutyric acid
KA	kainate
mAChR	muscarinic acetylcholine receptor
MEM	minimal essential medium
mGluR	metabotropic glutamate receptor
nAChR	nicotinergic acetylcholine receptor
NAD(P)H	nicotinamide adenine dinucleotide (phosphate)
NMDA	N-methyl-D-aspartate
NNT	nicotinamide nucleotide transhydrogenase
OHSC	organotypic hippocampal slice culture
PFA	paraformaldehyd
pO2	partial oxygen pressure
ROI	region of interest
ROT	rotenone
SLE	seizure-like event
SP	stratum pyramidale
SR	stratum radiatum
TCA cycle	tricarboxylic acid cycle

1 Introduction

1.1 Neuronal activity in the hippocampus

The hippocampus has become one of the most extensively studied areas of the mammalian brain and its proper function is of great importance, particularly for learning and memory. The hippocampus is involved in spatial navigation and the formation of declarative memory, which is defined as memory for facts (semantic memory) and events (episodic memory) (O'Keefe, 1979; Lopes da Silva et al., 1990). Therefore the hippocampus has to undergo constant changes. The ability of synaptic plasticity provides a basis for strong long-term potentiation (LTP) responses within the hippocampus, which are described as increases in the efficacy of synaptic transmission (Lopes da Silva et al., 1990). The hippocampus is also involved in the generation of epileptic seizures (Friedman et al., 2007) and it is known that the hippocampus is highly sensitive to damage which can result from e.g. temporal lope epilepsy, oxygen (O_2) starvation (anoxia) or encephalitis that often lead to major functional disturbance (Holopainen, 2005).

The hippocampus is characterized by its distinct laminated structure and its connections are largely unidirectional (see Fig. 3; Materials and Methods, page 18) (Witter and Amaral, 2004). The hippocampal input from the entorhinal cortex (layer II neurons) enters the dentate gyrus via the perforant path. Additionally, deep layer (IV-IV) neurons from the entorhinal cortex also project to the dentate gyrus and hippocampus (Heinemann et al., 2000). The main principal cells of the dentate gyrus are the granule cells in stratum granulosum. Their axons, the mossy fibres, project to stratum lucidum of area CA3 (cornu ammonis 3), where they form giant boutons, the characteristic mossy terminals, on the proximal dendrites of pyramidal cells. CA3 pyramidal cells have collateral projections to other CA3 pyramidal cells which terminate in stratum radiatum (SR) and stratum oriens. In addition, CA3 cells also receive a direct input from the entorhinal cortex, which innervates the most distal dendrites in stratum lacunosum moleculare. One major target of CA3 pyramidal cell axons, the schaffer collaterals, is the CA1 subfield. The main projections of CA1 pyramidal cells are to the subiculum and entorhinal cortex (Caeser and Aertsen, 1991). There is also a backpropagation from the entorhinal cortex (layer III neurons) directly into the subiculum and to CA1 (and

Introduction

probably to CA3 as well) where some pyramidal cells become activated, while most others are inhibited through feed-forward inhibition (Heinemann et al., 2000).
Beyond the principal cells of the hippocampus and dentate gyrus, there are various types of gamma-aminobutyric acid (GABA)ergic interneurons that provide inhibitory control of the excitatory loop (Freund and Buzsáki, 1996). The proportion of GABAergic neurons in the total neuronal population of the hippocampus has been studied by immunostainings of GABA and was found to be between 7% (Aika et al., 1994) and 11% (Woodson et al. 1989; Freund and Buzsáki, 1996). Interneurons of the hippocampus can be broadly classified by the innervation of spatially segregated domains on the somato-dendritic surface of principal cells (Gloveli et al., 2005). Thus, there are mainly two classes of interneurons, namely perisomatic targeting interneurons, such as basket and axo-axonic cells, and dendritic targetting cells, such as oriens lacunosum-moleculare (O-LM), bistratified and trilaminar interneurons (Gloveli et al., 2005). The heterogeneity of hippocampal interneurons is reflected in their synaptic mechanisms and firing patterns during different forms of neuronal network activity and thus they are suggested to play a major role in the generation of gamma oscillations (Freund and Buzsáki, 1996).

1.2 Gamma oscillations

Oscillatory activity occurs in several brain regions and refers to repetitive, almost periodic changes in the excitability or activity of single neurons or population of neurons (Whittington et al., 2000). Oscillatory activity of neuronal populations is also called network oscillations and is differentiated by frequencies between 0.005 to 500 Hz (Buzsáki and Draguhn, 2004). Different classes of oscillations are observed in different brain states and representing different behavioural correlates (Buzsáki and Draguhn, 2004). Frequencies from 0.5 up to 20 Hz are readily observable in electroencephalographic recordings during slow-wave sleep or relaxed wakefulness (Whittington et al., 2000; Fellous and Sejnowski, 2000). Frequencies from 4 to 10 Hz (theta oscillations) predominate during exploration and rapid eye movement (REM) sleep and are absent during slow-wave sleep. Fast oscillations in the gamma range (~30-80 Hz) can also be seen in the electroencephalographic signal but at much lower amplitudes during intense mental activity and following sensory stimulation (Whittington et al., 2000) and during REM sleep or exploration in the hippocampus of freely moving rats

(Fellous and Sejnowski, 2000), where they are superimposed on theta oscillations (Bragin et al., 1995; Whittington et al., 2000). Theta oscillations serve to modulate the amplitude of the faster gamma rhythm that, in turn, is thought to provide a temporal structure for higher brain functions, such as sensory processing, memory formation and perhaps consciousness (Buzsáki and Draguhn 2004; Bartos et al., 2007). Ultrafast oscillations (100-200 Hz), also called ripples, are present in rat hippocampus and parahippocampal regions and it is unknown whether a homologue exists in the human brain. However, ripples with higher frequencies (250-500 Hz) were observed in epileptogenic regions of patients with mesial temporal lobe epilepsie (Bragin et al., 1999).

Gamma oscillations were discovered by Freeman (Freeman 1959; 1978) in the olfactory bulb and periform cortex and they have been recorded in several other brain regions, such as somatosensory (MacDonald et al., 1996), auditory (Joliot et al., 1994) and visual cortices (Engel et al., 1991) and even in thalamic structures (Ribary et al., 1994) and in the hippocampus, where the power of the extracellularly recorded gamma oscillations is higher than in other brain regions, probably because of the laminated architecture of the hippocampal circuit (Förster et al., 2006). A major significance of gamma rhythm is that similar oscillations are simultaneously present in other forebrain areas during behavioural activation (Gray, 1994), therefore allowing the coupling of neocortical and hippocampal oscillations. This is a candidate mechanism for binding neuronal representations associated with currently perceived and retrieved information (Engel et al., 2001; Singer, 1993; Bragin et al., 1995; Buzsáki and Chrobak, 1995).

In vivo cholinergic septo-hippocampal fibres innervate principal neurons and interneurons of the hippocampus and thus have been discussed to have a possible pacemaker function in synchronizing hippocampal network activities (Stewart and Fox, 1990). Stimulation of this pathway has been shown to increase acetylcholine (ACh) levels in the hippocampus (Moroni et al., 1978). ACh acts on ionotropic nicotinergic ACh receptors (nAChR) and metabotropic muscarinic ACh receptors (mAChR). It is suggested that the oscillatory action of ACh is primarily mediated via mAChRs (Cobb and Davies, 2005) and that nAChRs do not participate in the genesis of oscillations *per se* but rather modulate pre-existing oscillatory states (Williams and Kauer, 1997; Cobb et al., 1999).

In hippocampal slice preparations the cholinergic input from the medial septal nucleus that provides the major source of cholinergic innervation to the hippocampus (Bartos et al., 2007;

Cobb and Davies, 2005) can be mimicked by bath application of ACh which induces gamma oscillations.

There are also other options to induce gamma oscillations in slice preparations, namely electrical stimulation, application of high potassium recording solution, application of kainate (KA) or metabotropic glutamate receptor agonists; these differ in the underlying cellular mechanisms (Pálhalmi et al., 2004; Bartos et al., 2007; Gloveli et al., 2005).

During cholinergic gamma oscillations both phasic inhibition from GABAergic interneurons and phasic excitation from glutamatergic pyramidal neurons are required (Bartos et al., 2007). Pyramidal neurons fire action potentials that are phase-related to the extracellular oscillation, but each neuron fires only during a small portion of the cycles (Fisahn et al., 1998) whereas fast-spiking interneurons like perisomatic targeting basket cells, bistratified cells and trilaminar interneurons discharge in a phase-locked manner to each gamma cycle (Bragin et al., 1995; Hájos et al., 2004; Gloveli et al., 2005), and thus are supposed to play an important role in generating gamma oscillations *in vitro* (Tukker et al., 2007). As a consequence, alternating pairs of current sinks and sources occur in stratum pyramidale (SP) and stratum radiatum (Csicsvari et al., 2003; Mann et al., 2005), which require enhanced activation of Na^+/K^+-ATPases to restore ionic gradients and to maintain excitability (Attwell and Iadecola, 2002). This leads to the suggestion that gamma oscillations might critically depend on sufficient supply of O_2 and glucose to maintain oxidative metabolism for the generation of adequate adenosine triphosphate (ATP). This is indirectly supported by a report showing that synchronized local field potential oscillations in the gamma range tightly correlate with hemodynamic signals *in vivo* (Niessing et al., 2005). Strikingly, the relationship between gamma oscillations and energy metabolism has been scarcely explored.

1.3 Oxidative energy metabolism in the brain

The brain accounts for 20% of the total O_2 consumption at rest, although it only constitutes of about 2% of the total body weight (Ndubuizu and LaManna, 2007; Rolfe and Brown, 1997) and it has very small energy stores, making neuronal activity and energy metabolism greatly dependent on constant O_2 and glucose delivery.

During glycolysis glucose is converted into pyruvate while nicotinamide adenine dinucleotide (NAD^+) is reduced to NADH and ATP is formed. Under anaerobic conditions pyruvate is

Introduction

converted into lactate in order to refuel the used NAD^+ pool and this could lead to an acidification of brain tissue. However, most of the ATP that is used in the brain is produced by oxidative phosphorylation and it requires sufficient glucose and O_2 availability (Erecinska and Silver, 2001). Therefore, brain mitochondria primarily utilize pyruvate from glycolysis to reduce nicotinamide adenine dinucleotides and flavin adenine dinucleotides (FAD) by enzymes of the tricarboxylic acid (TCA) cycle. While transforming electrons at the electron transport chain (ETC) from NADH and FAD to O_2, three of the four respiratory complexes (complex I, III and IV) extrude protons from the mitochondrial matrix (inner space) into the intermembrane space. This results in an inwardly directed proton gradient (ΔpH) across the inner mitochondrial membrane. The proton motive force is defined by ΔpH together with the mitochondrial membrane potential ($\Delta\Psi_m$) of 150 to 180 mV (negative with respect to cytosol) and it drives the mitochondrial ATP synthase (also known as F_oF_1 ATPase or complex V) to generate ATP (Kann and Kovács, 2007). It also generates a driving force for calcium (Ca^{2+}) ions in the matrix via the mitochondrial Ca^{2+} uniporter (Gunter et al., 2004; Mironov and Richter, 2001) (see Fig. 1). It was shown that in organotypic hippocampal slice cultures (OHSCs) Ca^{2+} is rapidly accumulated by the mitochondrion during neuronal activation (Kovács et al., 2001; 2005; Kann et al., 2005; 2003a; 2003b) Increases in the mitochondrial calcium concentration ($[Ca^{2+}]_m$) during neuronal activation, as well as the demand of ATP, regulate the activity of pyruvate dehydrogenase (which catalyzes the transformation of pyruvate to acetyl-CoA) and TCA cycle dehydrogenases (NAD^+-isocitrate dehydrogenases and α-ketogluterate dehydrogenases) and functionally modulate complexes IV and V (Hansford and Zorov, 1998; Kadenbach, 2003; McCormack et al., 1990).

To assure constant ATP production by mitochondrial oxidative phosphorylation, continuous supply of O_2 is essential to brain function. Disruption of O_2 delivery to the brain leads to loss of consciousness within seconds (Hansen, 1985) and decreases in O_2 availability cannot be tolerated for long periods because the energy supplied from anaerobic glycolysis is insufficient to maintain viability (Acker and Acker, 2004). Therefore, it is important to investigate the critical O_2 tension level at which homeostasis for cellular energetics and complex brain activities begins to fail. Early investigations with polarographic microelectrodes showed that the brain tissue's partial oxygen pressure (pO_2) can vary from ~90 mmHg very close to capillaries to much less than 34 mmHg in more distal regions (Zauner et. al, 2002) and the critical pO_2 for a breakdown of steady-state aerobic metabolism has been reported between 7 and 9 mmHg (Rolett et al., 2000). It is known that changes in

Introduction

tissue O_2 concentration reflect changes in blood-O_2 content and blood flow (Ndubuizu and LaManna, 2007) and it has been shown that changes in blood oxygenation *in vivo* could be detected with magnetic resonance imaging in rats (Ogawa et al., 1990) and in humans (Ogawa et al., 1992; Kwong et al., 1992). O_2 has to diffuse from the capillaries, which have an average distance of ~50-60 µm (Tata and Anderson, 2002; Zauner et al., 2002) in brain tissue and ultimately to mitochondria, where the oxidative phosphorylation takes place. It is speculated that neuronal mitochondria require an intracellular pO_2 of at least 1.5 mmHg to maintain aerobic metabolism (Verweij et al., 2007). O_2 tension in brain tissue varies within small distances and depends on the O_2 tension at the nearest capillary wall, the local tissue respiration, the diffusion coefficient for O_2 in the tissue and the distance from the capillary (Ndubuizu and LaManna, 2007). That explains why O_2 is heterogeneously distributed on a microregional level. Since *in vitro* slice preparations are separated from the vascular system, the tissue has to be supplied with O_2 from the bath solution by simple diffusion.

1.4 Monitoring of neuronal activity and mitochondrial redox state

To investigate the relationship between neuronal activity and mitochondrial redox state we used hippocampal slice preparations. Acute hippocampal slices have been reported to survive *in vitro* between 6 (Wang and Kass, 1997) and 24 hours (Djuricic et al., 1994). Organotypic slice cultures from young rats and mice (embryonic state up to postnatal day 16) can be kept alive for several weeks and they preserve the basic structural and connective organization of their tissue of origin. The term organotypic emphasizes the maintenance of characteristic properties unique to the type of tissue. According to the Stoppini method which was first described in 1991 (Stoppini et al., 1991), OHSCs are cultured up to 4 weeks on biopore membranes in interface conditions in an incubator (5% CO_2, 20% O_2, 36°C). Slice cultures are characterized by a well preserved multilayered organotypic organization, although they flatten to approximately 50% of the original thickness within a few days (Stoppini et al., 1991; Kann and Kovács, 2007) due to the degeneration of cells that had been damaged during the sectioning procedure. Slice cultures mature *in vitro* and synaptic reorganization occurs to a variable degree (Gutierrez and Heinemann, 1999) during the first week in culture, such as increased complexity of higher order dendritic branching and thus increased total number of synapses (De Simoni et al., 2003). Although connectivity is greater in OHSCs compared to

Introduction

acute slices development continues in both preparations at a remarkably similar rate once this is established and synaptic components like glutamate receptors are also maintained (Bahr et al., 1995).

Electrical stimuli to the fibre tracts from dentate gyrus to CA3 reveal neuronal activation in area CA3 that can be monitored with a K^+-sensitive microelectrode which gives us the opportunity to quantify the degree of neuronal activation. With this technique we are able to elicit temporally defined neuronal population responses, which are associated with characteristic NAD(P)H and FAD redox responses (Kann et al., 2005; Schuchmann et al., 2001; Foster et al., 2005). Since NADH and FAD are autofluorescent they can be easily used to monitor changes in mitochondrial redox state (Mayevsky and Chance, 1975; Schuchmann et al., 2001; Brennan et al. 2006; Kann et al., 2003a) and are therefore a useful tool to monitor mitochondrial energy metabolism. NADH and FAD autofluorescence has been first studied in isolated mitochondria (Chance et al., 1979) and later also in brain slice preparations and *in vivo* to monitor changes in cellular energy metabolism (Brennan et al., 2006; Kann et al., 2003a; 2003b; Mayevsky and Chance, 1975). When excited with ultraviolet light (340 nm and 360 nm, respectively) fluorescence emission with a maximal peak around 450 nm is attributed to the reduced forms, NADH and its phosphorylated form NADPH, while the oxidized forms (NAD^+ and $NADP^+$) are non-fluorescent (Aubin, 1979). The redox state of NADH and NADPH are coupled via the activity of the enzyme nicotin-amide nucleotide transhydrogenase (NNT), which is located at the inner mitochondrial membrane. As the emission spectra of NADH and NADPH overlap, NAD(P)H indicates that the recorded fluorescence might have originated from either one or both (Schuchmann et al., 2001). However, NADPH levels were found to be low in brain tissue (Chance et al., 1962; Kaplan, 1985; Klaidman et al., 2001). Changes in NAD(P)H fluorescence in brain slices are primarily due to activity of the mitochondrial ETC and the TCA cycle (Kann and Kovács, 2007). Under certain conditions, it might also be influenced by extramitochondrial signaling and antioxidative processes, where NADH and NADPH serve as cofactors (Berger et al., 2004; Dringen, 2000; Kirsch and de Groot, 2001). Moreover, in astrocytes with high glycolytic activity, occurring as a consequence of glutamate uptake, cytosolic NAD(P)H might significantly contribute to the overall NAD(P)H fluorescence (Kasischke et al., 2004).

After a period of excitatory stimulation brain slices usually show a decrease in NAD(P)H fluorescence, which is referred to as 'dip' component, followed by a much longer-lasting 'overshoot' component (Lipton, 1973; Schuchmann et al., 2001; Shuttleworth et al., 2003;

Introduction

Kasischke et al., 2004; Foster et al., 2005). The dip component reflects the oxidation phase; an acceleration of the ETC activity and the overshoot reflects the reduction phase; TCA cycle activity and glycolysis. Biphasic FAD transients (initial peak component and subsequent undershoot component) can be well matched to NAD(P)H transients, but of inverted sign (Brennan et al., 2006), because in this case the oxidized form is fluorescent. Although FAD fluorescence is weaker than NAD(P)H fluorescence, it has the advantage of an excitation maximum at 450 nm allowing prolonged recordings in brain slice preparations due to less phototoxicity (Kann and Kovács, 2007). Moreover, it has been reported that FAD fluorescence is more specific for mitochondria (Scholz et al., 1969; Kunz and Kunz, 1985; Huang et al., 2002).

To elucidate the specificity of mitochondrial function during gamma oscillations we applied rotenone, a high-affinity, specific inhibitor of the mitochondrial complex I (NADH dehydrogenase) of the ETC. Rotenone is a naturally occurring compound derived from the roots of certain plant species and it is a commonly used pesticide and insecticide (Betarbet et al., 2000; Alam and Schmidt, 2002). Since rotenone is extremely lipophilic it crosses biological membranes very rapidly (Alam and Schmidt, 2002) and thus has fast effects in slices.

Introduction

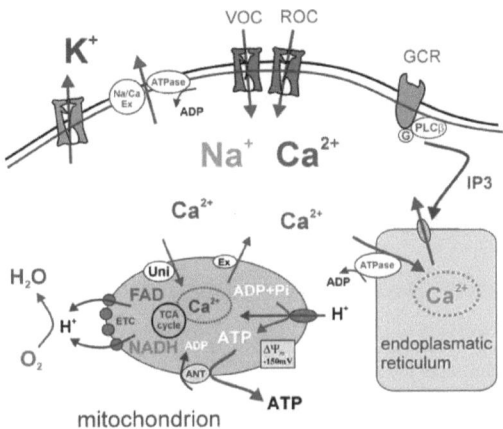

Figure 1. Neuronal activity and function of mitochondria.
Neuronal activity is associated with Ca^{2+} entry via voltage-operated channels (VOCs), receptor-operated channels (ROCs), store-operated channels (not shown), and nonselective cation channels (not shown), as well as Ca^{2+} release from endoplasmatic reticulum via receptors for inositol (1,4,5)-trisphosphate (IP3R) and ryanodine (not shown). Neuronal activation also causes accumulation of intracellular Na^+ and extracellular K^+. To maintain ionic gradients across the neuronal membrane, Na^+/K^+-ATPase and Ca^{2+}-ATPase consume large amounts of ATP. Mitochondria take up Ca^{2+} in the vicinity to sites of Ca^{2+} influx and/or Ca^{2+} release via the mitochondrial uniporter (Uni). Glycolysis and lactate dehydrogenase-1 (not shown) provide NADH and pyruvate that is transferred to the mitochondrial matrix and converted by pyruvate dehydrogenase complex (not shown) to fuel the tricarboxylic acid (TCA) cycle. NADH and FAD transfer energy from the TCA cycle to complex I and complex II of the ETC respectively. ETC activity leads to O_2 consumption and to a proton gradient across the inner mitochondrial membrane, which results in a proton motive force that leads to the production of ATP by the ATP synthase. Further abbreviations: ANT (adenine nucleotide translocase), GCR (G-protein coupled receptor), PCL (phospholipase C), Na/Ca Ex (Na^+/Ca^{2+} exchanger). (Modified from Kann and Kovács, 2007).

Since in acute hippocampal slices and also in OHSCs the tri-synaptic fibre pathway and the distinct laminated structure are maintained, they are both appropriate models for studying different forms of neuronal activity as evoked by electrical stimulation or intrinsic network oscillations. Compared to acute slices OHSCs have the advantages of lower diffusion distances for drugs, ions, and O_2 and the absence of a non-vital superficial layer which could act as an O_2 barrier (Lipinski, 1989). In both slice preparations changes in NAD(P)H and FAD autofluorescence can be used to monitor mitochondrial redox state and thus energy metabolism.

2 Aim of the study

Gamma oscillations are in the range of ~30-80 Hz and have been shown to play an important role in higher brain functions, such as learning and memory and perhaps consciousness (Buzsáki and Draguhn, 2004; Bartos et al., 2007). It has been demonstrated that O_2 availability is a key factor in processes which are related to this type of neuronal network oscillations, e.g. lowering O_2 concentration in the brain leads to an impaired ability to perform complex tasks and further decreases results in impaired short-term memory and loss of consciousness (Verweij et al., 2007). Thus we hypothesized that gamma oscillations are highly dependent on adequate O_2 supply.

The first aim of this study was to investigate the sensitivity of gamma oscillations to pO_2 decreases in the CA3 subfield of hippocampal slice preparations.

In the CA3 subfield of the hippocampus gamma oscillations arise from the precise interplay of action potential firing of excitatory glutamatergic principal neurons and fast inhibitory GABAergic interneurons. As a consequence, alternating pairs of current sinks and sources occur in stratum pyramidale and stratum radiatum, which require enhanced activation of Na^+/K^+-ATPases to restore ionic gradients and to maintain excitability. Hence, we hypothesized that gamma oscillations might critically depend on sufficient neuronal ATP supply and thus proper mitochondrial function. This is indirectly supported by a report showing that synchronized gamma oscillations and hemodynamic signals tightly correlate *in vivo* (Niessing et al., 2005).

The second aim of this study was to determine the oxygen consumption and functional performance of mitochondria during gamma oscillations.

We have to emphasize that the fundamental relationships between gamma oscillations, mitochondrial function and O_2 consumption have not been defined.

Aim of the study

Specific aims were to:
1. establish an *in vitro* model for gamma oscillations in acute mouse hippocampal slices and in rat OHSCs
2. determine the sensitivity of gamma oscillations to decreases in tissue pO_2 in relation to other forms of neuronal activity
3. measure the O_2 consumption during gamma oscillations
4. examine the mitochondrial redox state during gamma oscillations by monitoring NAD(P)H and FAD fluorescence
5. elucidate the role of mitochondrial performance during gamma oscillations by applying rotenone, a lipophilic and specific inhibitor of the mitochondrial complex I of the ETC
6. establish an *in vitro* model for chronic complex I inhibition with rotenone.

To test our hypotheses we studied mitochondrial function and O_2 consumption during gamma oscillations either in acute mouse hippocampal slices or in rat OHSCs. Gamma oscillations in hippocampal slice preparations can be evoked by ACh which mimics cholinergic input from the septum and they share many features with physiological gamma oscillations *in vivo* (Bragin et al., 1995; Csicsvari et al., 2003).

Using electrophysiology, O_2 sensor microelectrode and imaging techniques, we investigated the interactions of neuronal network activity, tissue pO_2 and mitochondrial redox state in the CA3 subfield of hippocampal slice preparations.

This project reveals the importance of proper mitochondria function during fast neuronal network oscillations and it addresses the question whether mitochondrial dysfunction acts as a critical factor for the vulnerability of complex brain functions that might occur during aging, ischemia, neurodegenerative and psychiatric diseases.

3 Materials and Methods

3.1 Organotypic hippocampal slice cultures (OHSCs)

OHSCs were prepared using the Stoppini method (Stoppini et al. 1991; Kann et al., 2003a; 2003b) (Fig. 2). The brain from 7- to 9-days-old wistar rat was removed and the hemispheres were separated. Both hippocampi were detached with a small spatula from the occipital and rostral sides and were positioned on a filter paper moisturized with cold minimal essential medium (MEM, Gibco, Invitrogen, Karlsruhe, Germany; No. 11012-044). Hippocampi, still attached to the filter paper, were transferred to a tissue chopper (McIlwain, Mickle Laboratory, Gomshall, Surrey, England) and were cut in 400 μm thick slices along the longitudinal axis under sterile conditions. Slices were rinsed with medium and were collected in cold MEM saturated with 95% O_2 and 5% CO_2. Slices were maintained on a biomembrane surface (Millipore, Eschborn, Germany) between culture medium (50 % MEM, 25 % Hank's balanced salt solution (Sigma-Aldrich, Taufkirchen, Germany), 25 % horse serum (Gibco) and 2 mM L-glutamine (Gibco) at pH 7.3) and humidified atmosphere (5 % CO_2, 36.5° C) in an incubator (Unitherm 150, UniEquip, Martinsried, Germany).

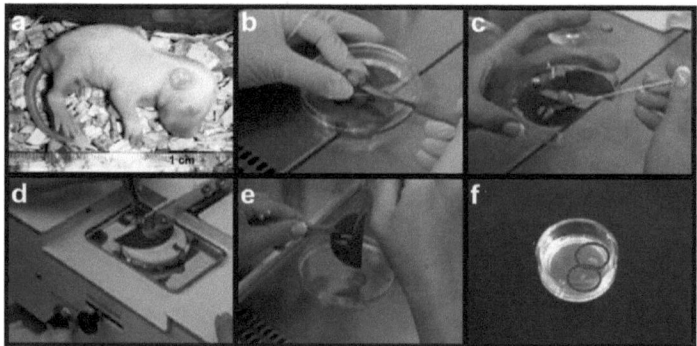

Figure 2. Preparation of rat OHSCs.
Preparation of OHSCs from 7-days-old wistar rat (**a**). The brain was removed (**b**), hippocampi were isolated (**c**) and cut with a tissue chopper (**d**) in 400 μm thick slices. Slices were rinsed with MEM (**e**) and collected on a biomembrane surface (**f**) between culture medium.

Materials and Methods

The transparent biomembrane has no autofluorescence and can thus be used for fluorescence imaging procedures (Stoppini et al., 1991).
Half of the medium was replaced three times per week. Slice cultures were used for experiments between 7 and 17 days *in vitro* (*div*) (residual thickness of 180-210 µm).

3.2 Acute hippocampal slices

Acute hippocampal slices were prepared from brains of 20 to 30 day old C57BL/6 mice. Mice were decapitated under deep isoflurane (forene, active agent: isoflurane, Abbott GmbH, Wiesbaden, Germany) anaesthesia. Their brains were rapidly removed and immersed in ice-cold and carbogenated artificial cerebrospinal fluid (ACSF). The brain was placed on filter tissue soaked with ice-cold ACSF and the cerebellum was removed with a scalpel. The two hemispheres were separated and were glued with the dorsal site on a cold cutting block immersed in cold ACSF. Horizontal hippocampal slices (400 µm) were cut with a vibratome (Leica VT 1000S, Leica Microsystems, Nussloch, Germany) from the ventral and dorsal hippocampus and were immediately transferred into an interface-type recording chamber continuously perfused with warm ACSF (34±0.5 °C, flow rate 2 ml/min, pH 7.4). Slices were stored for at least 1.5 hours before performing experiments.
Animal procedures were conducted in accordance with the guidelines of the European Communities Council and approved by the Berlin Animal Ethics Committee (T0291/04 and T0032/08).

3.3 Solutions and recordings

Acute mouse hippocampal slices or rat OHSCs on excised membranes were maintained in the recording chamber with saturated (20% or 95% O_2, 5% CO_2) ACSF that contained in mM: NaCl 129, KCl 3, NaH_2PO_4 1.25, $MgSO_4$ 1.8, $CaCl_2$ 1.6, $NaHCO_3$ 21 and glucose 10 (pH 7.3). Components of ACSF were from Sigma-Aldrich.
Experiments were performed at 34±1° C in an interface chamber or at 24-26 °C under submerged recording conditions with ACSF flow rates of 2 and 5 ml/min, respectively. Fluorescence and accompanying pO_2 recordings were made under submerged conditions with

Materials and Methods

recording chambers mounted on either an upright Axioskop (Zeiss, Jena, Germany) or a BX51WI microscope (Olympus, Hamburg, Germany) using 20x (0.5 numerical aperture (NA)) and 10x (0.3 NA) water immersion objectives or a 4x objective (0.28 NA) with a water cap.

For recordings of gamma oscillations, either submerged recording chambers or self-made interface recording chambers, which allow rapid exchange of the gas atmosphere (Hoffmann et al., 2006), were used. For induction of gamma oscillations 5 to 10 µM ACh and 1 to 2 µM Physostigmine (submerged recording conditions) and 2 µM ACh and 400 nM Physostigmine (interface recording conditions) were used, respectively. ACh was from Sigma-Aldrich, Physostigmine was from Tocris (Biotrend, Köln, Germany).

To inhibit the complex I of the ETC the specific inhibitor rotenone was used (Sigma-Aldrich).

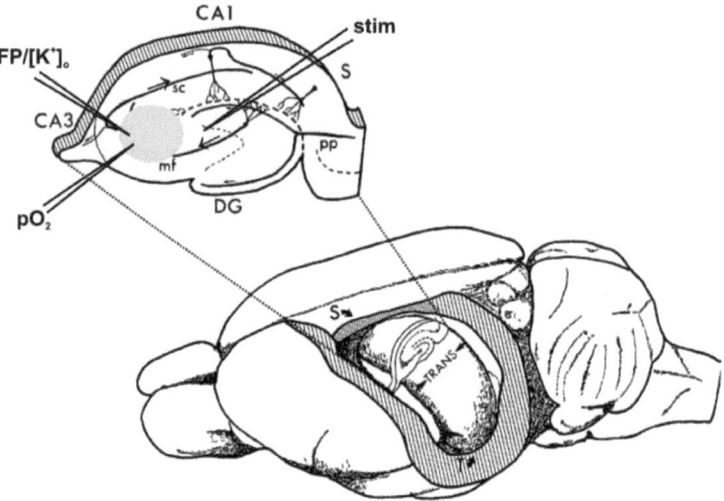

Figure 3. Line drawing of the hippocampal formation and its position within the rat brain.
The activity enters the dentate gyrus (**DG**) by the perforant path (**pp**) and is transmitted along the mossy fibres (**mf**) to area CA3 and runs further along the schaffer collaterals (**sc**) to area CA1 and opens to the subiculum (**S**). Arrows indicate electrophysiological tools which were applied in different experimental procedures. Electrical stimulation (**stim**) led to changes in NAD(P)H and FAD fluorescence (solid grey circle). Extracellular field potentials (**FP**) and changes in $[K^+]_o$ were monitored in area CA3 as well as changes in tissue oxygenation (**pO₂**).
(Modified from Andersen et al., 2007).

Materials and Methods

Recording microelectrodes (K^+-sensitive/field potential, O_2-sensitive) were placed in stratum pyramidale of area CA3. Multiple unit activity was recorded with low impedance tungsten in glass microelectrodes and single units were discriminated with a template matching algorithm (Gaedicke and Albus, 1995) in recording periods of 180 s.

Field potentials and changes in extracellular potassium were recorded with a K^+-sensitive microelectrode (Heinemann and Arens, 1992), which consists of double-barreled theta glass (Science Products, Hofheim, Germany). The reference barrel was filled with 154 mM NaCl solution, the ion-sensitive barrel with potassium ionophore I cocktail A (60031, Fluka Chemie, Buchs, Switzerland) and 100 mM KCl. K^+-sensitive microelectrodes with a sensitivity of 58 ± 2 mV to a tenfold increase in $[K^+]$ were used for experiments. The amplifier was equipped with negative capacitance feedback control, which permitted recordings of changes in $[K^+]_o$ with time constants of <50 to 200 ms. Changes in voltage were digitised at 10 Hz (and low pass filtered at 3 kHz) using CED 1401 interface and Spike 2 software (Cambridge Electronic Design, Cambrigde, UK) or FeliX software (Photon Technology Instruments, Wedel, Germany).

Evoked local field potential responses elicited by single electrical stimuli (0.1 ms duration) to the fibre tracts from dentate gyrus to CA3, and neuronal activation evoked by electrical stimulus trains (10 s at 20 Hz or 1 s at 100 Hz) (see Fig. 3) were induced either by bipolar tungsten in glass microelectrodes (self-manufactured, tungsten filament with a tip diameter of 5-15 μm) or monopolar glass electrodes (Science Products, Hofheim, Germany) filled with ACSF.

3.4 O_2-sensitive microelectrode

Clark-style glass O_2 microelectrodes (tip diameter of 10 μm, either from Diamond General Development, Ann Arbor, MI, USA, No. 737GC or from Unisense, Aarhus, Denmark, No. OX10) were used to continuously measure changes in pO_2. This new type of modified Clark electrode has the advantages of low sensitivity to motion artefact, a time constant of <1 s (0-90%), minimal interaction with tissue and low O_2 consumption (Foster et al., 2005; Pomper et al., 2006; Takano et al., 2007). The O_2 sensor consists of a gold-coated sensing cathode which is polarized against the internal Ag/AgCl reference anode. Additionally, an internal silver wire guard cathode, which is polarized, scavenges O_2 in the electrolyte (KCl) within the electrode, thus minimizing zero-current and pre-polarization time. Driven by the external partial pressure, O_2 from the environment penetrates through the sensor tip membrane and is reduced at the gold cathode surface, resulting in a current flow. The reaction at the sensing cathode is expressed as:

$$O_2 + 2\ H_2O + 4\ e^- \rightarrow 4\ OH^-$$

The reaction at the Ag/AgCl reference anode is expressed as:

$$4\ Ag + 4\ Cl^- \rightarrow 4\ AgCl + 4\ e^-$$

For polarization, the electrode was connected to a polarographic amplifier (Chemical Microsensor II, Diamond General) and the tip was maintained in non-gassed ACSF overnight. The O_2 sensor was polarized with -0.80 V which resulted in a stable current readout. Before and after each experiment, the electrode was calibrated by generating a three-point calibration curve in ACSF saturated with 100% N_2, 20% O_2 (5% CO_2, 75% N_2) or 95% O_2 (5% CO_2) at stable temperature, which revealed a linear relationship between current readout and pO_2. For experiments, the polarographic amplifier that provides an analogous output signal which is proportional to the polarographic current was connected to the data acquisition unit (CED Micro 1401 interface). The O_2 sensor was placed closely to the K^+-sensitive/field potential recording electrode in CA3. Changes in voltage from both electrodes were low pass filtered and simultaneously digitized at 1 and 5 (field potential) kHz.

3.5 Fluorescence recordings of NAD(P)H and FAD

Nicotinamide adenine dinucleotide (phosphate) (NAD(P)H) and flavin adenosine dinucleotide (FAD) were excited at 360±15 nm (or 720 nm) and 490±10 nm, respectively. Recordings were made with a monochromator system (Photon Technology Instruments, Wedel, Germany) or with a 2-photon fluorescence microscope (Leica TCS SP2, Leica Microsystems, Wetzlar, Germany) or with an epifluorescence illumination system (Olympus Cell^R) that combines a fast driven excitation filter wheel and a triple band emission filter, allowing almost simultaneous excitation of NAD(P)H and FAD (delay ~130 ms). NAD(P)H and FAD fluorescence images (emission at 460±10 nm and 530±10 nm, respectively) were recorded at 0.5 Hz using a CCD camera (ORCA-ER, Hamamatsu Photonics, Hamamatsu City, Japan)

Materials and Methods

connected to Cell^R system and software (Olympus BioSystems GmbH, Planegg, Germany). Fast NAD(P)H fluorescence recordings were made at 10 Hz using photomultiplier-based microfluorimetry (Seefelder Messtechnik, Seefeld, Germany) and FeliX software (Photon Technology Instruments). Changes in NAD(P)H and FAD fluorescence are presented as changes in %$\Delta F/F_0$ ($\Delta F/F_0 *100$) where F_0 is the averaged fluorescence of a 20 s period before electrical or chemical stimulation of the tissue.

3.6 Fluorescence recordings of rhodamine-123

To measure relative changes of mitochondrial membrane potential ($\Delta\Psi$), we used the fluorescent dye rhodamine-123 (Sigma-Aldrich). The permeant dye accumulates in polarized intracellular compartments such as mitochondria (Duchen, 1992). At appropriate concentrations, the accumulated dye will self-quench, thereby reducing its quantum yield. A depolarizing change of $\Delta\Psi$ is indicated by an increase in rhodamine fluorescence signal in response to dequenching of the dye after release from mitochondria.

For high spatial resolution images of mitochondria, slice cultures were stained with 5 µM rhodamine-123 (excitation: 490±10 nm, emission: 530±10 nm) for 10 min and images were acquired with a 2-photon fluorescence microscope (Leica TCS SP2, Leica Microsystems, Wetzlar, Germany).

3.7 Chronic rotenone treatment of OHSCs and Fluoro-Jade B staining

Fluoro-Jade B (FJB) was used to study neuronal degeneration after chronic treatment of OHSCs with the complex I inhibitor rotenone. FJB is a polyanionic fluorescein derivative with an excitation peak at 480 nm, and an emission peak at 525 nm and it stains degenerating neurons and their processes regardless of the mechanism by which a neuron dies (Schmued and Hopkins, 2000). OHSCs were treated with 10, 20 and 50 nM rotenone from 3 to 8 *div* after preparation. Rotenone was applied to the culture medium, which was replaced completely at day 3 and day 6. As 100% controls slice cultures were incubated with 5 µM N-

Materials and Methods

Methyl-D-Aspartat (NMDA) (Tocris, Biozol Vertrieb GmbH, Eching, Germany) and 5 µM KA (Tocris, Biozol) for 24 h before they were fixated.

At day 8 the slice cultures, still attached to the membrane, were either used for combined electrophysiological and NAD(P)H/FAD fluorescence measurements or were fixed with 4% paraformaldehyde (PFA) and 0.5% glutaraledehyde (Carl Roth GmbH, Karlsruhe, Germany) for at least 24 h at 4°C for staining procedure. Before cutting the fixed OHSCs with a freezing microtome (rotary microtome and freezing device from Leica, Wetzlar, Germany) in slices of 30 µm thickness, they were immersed in a sucrose solution (30% sucrose in 0.01 PB) over night at 4°C. Sections were mounted on gelatine coated glass slides and were dried before staining. During the staining procedure the slices remained on the glass slides and were immersed in ethyl alcohol containing 25% NaOH (Roth) for 5 min, followed by 2 min of 70% ethanol and were washed for 2 min with distilled water. After rehydration slides were transferred to 0.06% potassium permanganate (Fluka, Sigma-Aldrich, Steinheim, Germany) for 10 min, washed with distilled water for 2 min and were than transferred to the FJB solution (Histo-Chem Inc., Jefferson, AR, USA) for 20 min. A 0.01% stock solution of the dye was prepared by dissolving 10 mg FJB in 100 ml of distilled water. 10 ml of the stock solution were added to 90 ml of 0.1% acetic acid (VWR International GmbH, Darmstadt, Germany) in distilled water to obtain the usable FJB solution of 0.001%. After staining the sections were rinsed three times with distilled water. Excess water was drained off, and the slides were dried on a heating plate and coverslipped with Entellan (VWR). For the examination of FJB-positive cells in rotenone-treated OHSCs, a microscope connected to an epifluorescence illumination system (Cell^R, Olympus, Hamburg, Germany) equipped with a FITC filter system and a CCD camera (ORCA-ER, Hamamatsu Photonics, Hamamatsu City, Japan) was used. Images were taken with a 20x objective and were saved for further analysis. In each image a rectangle of 100 µm x 300 µm was positioned over the cell layer in each of the following regions: CA1, CA2, CA3, dentate gyrus. Within the defined rectangle all FJB-positive cells were counted by eye performed by two observers independently (there was no significant difference between the two observers), and a mean value was calculated. Statistical significance was determined and histograms were performed with Origin (Microcal Software, Northamton, MA).

3.8 Calculations and statistics

To translate the recorded potential values (mV) in $[K^+]_o$, a modified Nernst equation was used:

Equation: $\log[\text{Ion}]_1 = E_M * (s * v)^{-1} + \log[\text{Ion}]_o$,

with E_M, recorded potential; s, electrode slope obtained at calibration; v, valence of the specific ion; $[\text{Ion}]_o$, ion concentration at rest; and $[\text{Ion}]_1$, ion concentration during activation.

Power spectra of fast network oscillations were calculated by fast Fourier transformation (FFT size 1024, Hanning window) for three data segments of 60 s each: 1) at 95% O_2 gassing (control condition), 2) after 2 min at 20% O_2, 3) after 2 min at 95% O_2 (reoxygenation). For comparison of power spectra at 20% O_2 and reoxygenation, the sum of the power of the bins from 30–80 Hz was calculated and normalized to the control condition. In an additional set of experiments (see Fig. 4 and Fig. 5) power spectra as well as auto- and cross-correlograms were calculated from data segments of 120 s. Powers spectra were approximated with a single Gaussian fit. Parameters of the Gaussian fit (r^2, height, area under the curve and full width at half maximum (FWHM)) were normalized and tested on statistical significance by using paired t-test. For analysis of gamma oscillations, data were filtered at 0.2 kHz offline (Fisahn et al., 1998).

Data are reported as mean ± standard error (SE) and are derived from at least three slice culture preparations per experimental group. Statistical significance ($p<0.05$) was determined using Student's *t*-tests and ANOVA (Friedman's test and Dunn's posthoc test). Calculations and figures were made using Spike 2 (Cambridge Electronic Design), Clampfit 9 (Axon Instruments, Union City, CA, USA), Origin (Microcal Software, Northampton, MA, USA) and CorelDRAW (Corel Corporation, Ottawa, Ontario, Canada).

4 Results

4.1 Gamma oscillations in rat OHSCs and acute mouse hippocampal slices induced by acetylcholine

Permanent bath application of ACh (in the presence of the cholinesterase inhibitor physostigmine) resulted in robust gamma oscillations in both CA3 and CA1 of acute mouse hippocampal slices (Fig. 4) and in rat OHSCs (Fig. 5). To verify the *in vitro* model for gamma oscillations atropine, a competitive muscarinic ACh receptor antagonist was applied during persistent gamma oscillations. Atropine totally abolished gamma oscillations in acute mouse slices (Fig. 4C) and thus shows that gamma oscillations depend on muscarinic ACh receptor activation. In contrast to CA3 and CA1, gamma oscillations were absent in the dentate gyrus in acute slices (Fig. 4A) and OHSCs (not shown). Highest amplitudes of oscillations were observed in the distal part of CA3 compared to the proximal part (not shown) and CA1. In auto-correlograms, the leading peak frequencies (39 Hz in acute slices and 41 Hz in OHSCs) of gamma oscillations did not differ in CA3 and CA1 (Table 1). Cross-correlograms showed a high synchrony between oscillations in area CA3 and CA1 (coefficients of 0.62±0.06, n=4 in acute slices and 0.58±0.03, n=5 in OHSCs) and a phase lag of 1.0±0.05 ms (n=4) and 1.19±0.1 ms (n=5), respectively, indicating propagation of the activity from CA3 to CA1. Fast Fourier transform algorithms revealed high power of oscillations in bins from 30 to 60 Hz in both subfields in acute slices (Fig. 4B), and also in OHSCs in bins of 25-45 Hz. Each power spectrum in this range was approximated with a single Gaussian fit. Area and height of the fits were significantly greater in CA3 (Table 1), clearly demonstrating a higher power of gamma oscillations. FWHM did not differ in both subfields (Table 1).

These data show that gamma oscillations are consistently more prominent in area CA3 and propagate to area CA1 in acute mouse hippocampal slices and rat OHSCs. Similar characteristics of hippocampal gamma oscillations have been reported from acute rat hippocampal slices (Fisahn et al., 1998; Wójtowicz et al., 2009) and *in vivo* (Bragin et al., 1995). Consequently, both acute mouse hippocampal slices and rat OHSCs are appropriate models to study cholinergic gamma oscillations *in vitro*.

Results

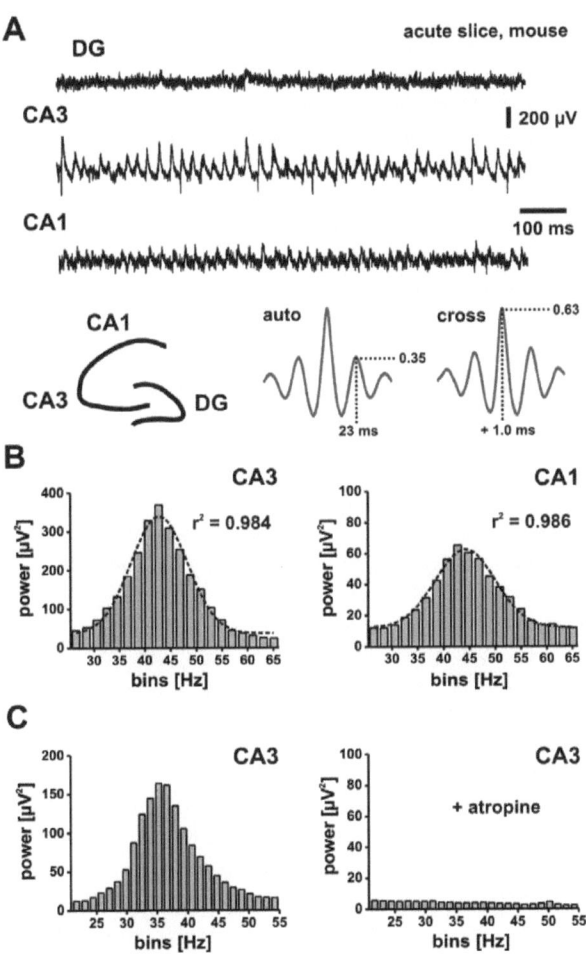

Figure 4. Gamma oscillations in acute mouse hippocampal slices.

(A) Local field potential recordings (traces) were made in the presence of ACh (2 µM) and physostigmine (400 nM) in CA3, CA1 and dentate gyrus (DG, scheme) of acute slices. Note that robust and persistent gamma oscillations were more prominent in CA3 compared with CA1 and absent in the dentate gyrus. The CA3 auto-correlogram (auto) revealed a leading peak frequency of gamma oscillations of 43 Hz. The cross-correlogram (cross) revealed a phase lag of 1 ms for oscillations in CA1 (with reference to CA3). (B) Power spectra were precisely approximated with a single Gaussian fit (see Table 1). Note that the power of gamma oscillations was greater in CA3 (scaling of ordinates). (C) Representative power spectra illustrating that bath application of atropine (1 µM) completely blocked robust and persistent gamma oscillations (n=4). Recordings were made under interface conditions.

Results

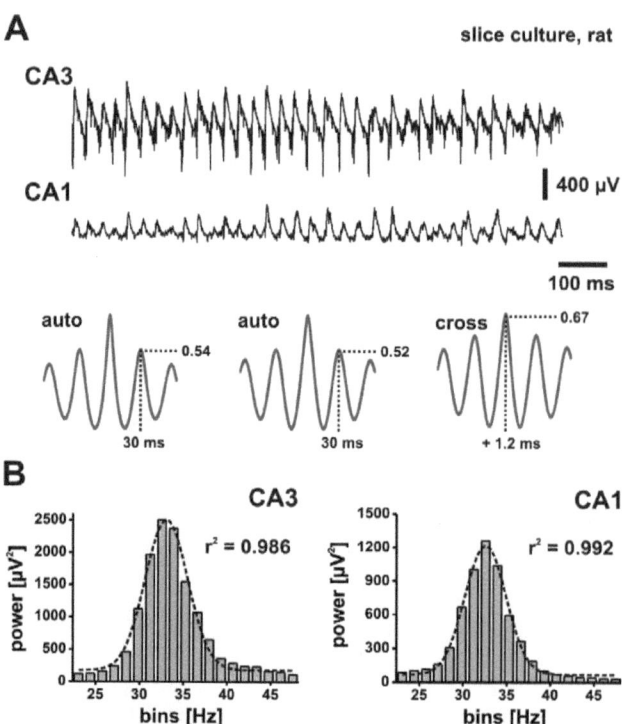

Figure 5. Gamma oscillations in rat OHSCs.

(A) Local field potential recordings were made in the presence of ACh (2 µM) and physostigmine (400 nM) in CA3 and CA1 (traces) of rat OHSCs. Auto-correlograms (auto) revealed a leading peak frequency of gamma oscillations of 33 Hz in both CA3 (left) and CA1 (middle). The cross-correlogram (cross, right) revealed a phase lag of 1.2 ms for oscillations in CA1 (with reference to CA3). (B) Power spectra were precisely approximated with a single Gaussian fit (see Table 1). Note that the power of gamma oscillations was greater in CA3 (scaling of ordinates). Recordings were made under interface conditions.

Results

mouse	CA3	CA1	n	p-value
lpf*	39.3 ± 1.2	39.8 ± 1.2	9	0.12
acc*	0.42 ± 0.03	0.26 ± 0.02	9	<0.01
r^2	0.985 ± 0.002	0.975 ± 0.006	9	0.10
FWHM	10.45 ± 0.76	10.71 ± 0.80	9	0.17
A	5911 ± 1046	994 ± 223	9	<0.01
H	592 ± 142	84 ± 18	9	<0.01

rat	CA3	CA1	n	p-value
lpf*	41.6 ± 3.0	41.3 ± 2.9	7	0.74
acc*	0.39 ± 0.04	0.37 ± 0.03	7	0.31
r^2	0.985 ± 0.003	0.982 ± 0.004	7	0.53
FWHM	12.55 ± 1.90	12.15 ± 1.82	7	0.31
A	11457 ± 1102	4475 ± 1230	7	<0.01
H	1115 ± 296	469 ± 171	7	<0.01

<u>**Table 1.**</u> **Results from auto-correlograms (*) (Figures 4A, 5A) and single Gaussian fits (Figures 4B, 5B).**

Abbreviations and units: leading peak frequency (**lpf**; Hz), auto-correlation coefficient (**acc**), correlation coefficient (r^2), full width at half maximum (**FWHM**; Hz), area (**A**; $\mu V^2 * Hz$) and height (**H**; μV^2). Note that area and height are significantly greater in area CA3 in both acute mouse hippocampal slices (upper part) and rat OHSCs (lower part).

Results

4.2 Neuronal activity and its sensitivity to decreases in tissue pO_2

To study the O_2 dependence of cholinergic gamma oscillations in area CA3 we determined changes of local field potentials during decreases of tissue oxygenation within the norm-oxic range. To compare the effects of decreases of tissue oxygenation on gamma oscillations we also looked at other forms of neuronal activity, namely spontaneous network activity and evoked local field potential responses, and their sensitivity to tissue pO_2. For this set of experiments we used rat OHSCs.

4.2.1 Gamma oscillations

Gamma oscillations in stratum pyramidale in area CA3 of rat OHSCs were evoked by bath application of ACh in the presence of cholinesterase inhibitor physostigmine under interface and also under submerged recording conditions. Under submerged recording conditions fluorescence measurements could be performed. Gamma oscillations were persistent up to hours and the highest power was observed in bins of 45-50 Hz (Fig. 6). After a switch from 95% O_2 to 20% O_2 the gamma band power (30-80 Hz) was significantly reduced after 1-2 min (Fig. 6A, traces, and corresponding power spectra in 6B, $p<0.001$, $n=15$). Switching back to 95% O_2 led to a full recovery of gamma oscillations, whereas in some experiments gamma oscillations showed a higher power within the first 2-5 min during reoxygenation. However, this effect was not statistically significant when compared with the 95% O_2 control condition ($n=15$, $p=0.49$).

Results

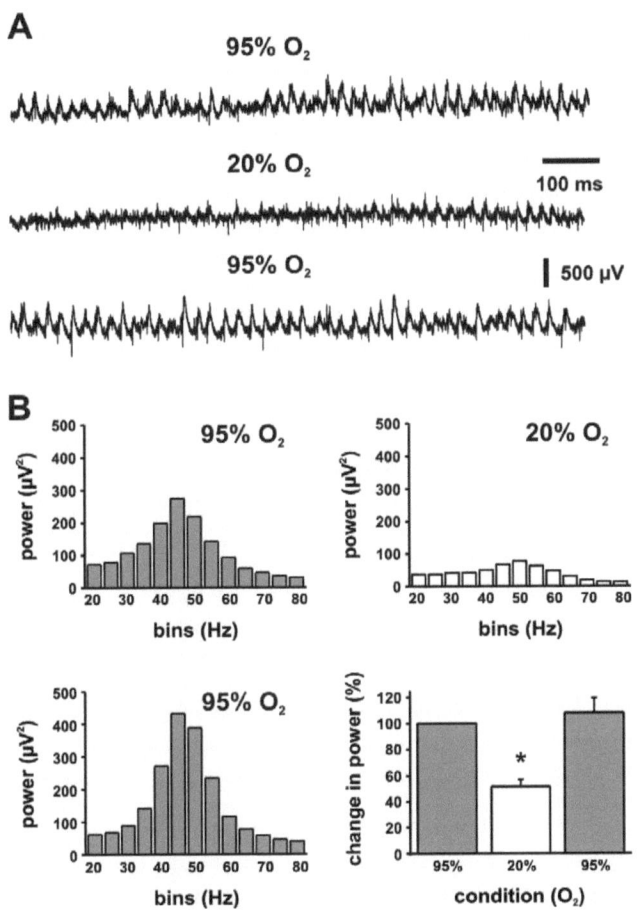

Figure 6. Effects of tissue oxygenation on cholinergic gamma oscillations.

(A) Local field potential responses were recorded in SP, and ACh was continuously applied in the presence of cholinesterase inhibitor physostigmine to evoke robust and persistent gamma oscillations. (B) From recordings and conditions as illustrated in A, power spectra were calculated from data segments of 60 s. Recordings were made in area CA3 of rat OHSCs under interface conditions. *p<0.05

Results

4.2.2 Spontaneous network activity and evoked local field potential responses

To test whether the sensitivity to decreases in pO_2 was specific for gamma oscillations, we also determined the effects of tissue oxygenation on spontaneous network activity and evoked local field potential responses.
By using multiunit recordings in area CA3 of rat OHSCs, we found that spontaneous network activity decreased within minutes at 20% O_2 (Fig. 7A). To get further insight into the characteristics of the neurons that were affected, we discriminated single units during 180 min of stable recordings at 95% O_2, and classified them according to spike-rates in three groups, showing <2, 2-5, and >5 spikes per second, respectively (Fig. 7B). At 20% O_2, the spike rates decreased in all groups and reversed completely during reoxygenation. The strongest spike reduction occurred after 30-60 min at 20% O_2.
In sharp contrast to spontaneous network activity and cholinergic gamma oscillations, shape and amplitude (1.7±0.1 mV versus 1.8±0.1 mV, n=10, p=0.49) of local field potential responses as elicited by moderate electrical stimuli were unaffected by changes in tissue oxygenation (Fig. 7C).

These data indicated that specifically gamma oscillations and spontaneous network activity were highly sensitive to decreases in tissue pO_2, which might have been mediated by limitations of O_2 availability during 20% O_2. Therefore, we quantified the interstitial pO_2 in the slice core of rat OHSCs during 20% and 95% O_2. Additionally, we monitored changes in NAD(P)H fluorescence which reflects changes in mitochondrial redox state during low and high pO_2. By applying O_2 sensor microelectrode and monitoring NAD(P)H and FAD fluorescence during defined neuronal stimulation responses, we next tested whether O_2 consumption and mitochondrial redox state differ in both oxygenation conditions.

Results

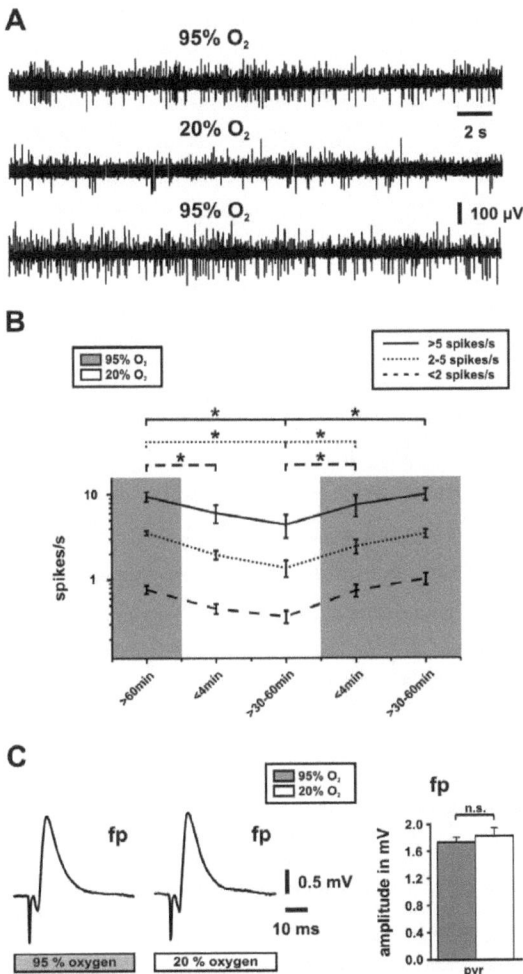

Figure 7. Effects of tissue oxygenation on spontaneous network activity and evoked local field potential responses.

(A) Multiunit activity was recorded continuously in SP, and oxygenation was changed according to the protocol as illustrated in B. (B) Single-unit discrimination in recording periods of 180 s. Single units were classified in three groups according to their spike rates (spike/s), which revealed a distribution of 10% (solid line), 22% (dotted line), and 68% (dashed line) (from n=69) at 95% O_2 (grey background). Note that the spike rates declined in all groups at 20% O_2 (white background), which was reversible. (C) After 15 min under the respective oxygenation condition, local field potentials were evoked orthodromically by application of single electrical stimuli to the fibre tracts from dentate gyrus to area CA3. Note that there were no differences in shape and amplitude of the responses. Recordings were made in area CA3 of rat OHSCs under submerged conditions. *$p<0.05$

Results

4.3 Changes in interstitial pO_2 and mitochondrial redox state

To quantify interstitial pO_2 levels and changes in mitochondrial redox state under both oxygenation conditions we used Clark-style O_2 sensor microelectrodes that have been commonly used to monitor interstitial pO_2 levels in hippocampal slice preparations (Foster et al., 2005; Pomper et al., 2006; Huchzermeyer et al., 2008) and in the brain *in vivo* (Offenhauser et al., 2005; Takano et al., 2007), and fluorescence recordings of NAD(P)H and FAD.

Because gamma oscillations were highly sensitive to decreases in tissue pO_2 and elicited only slow elevations in NAD(P)H fluorescence under the 95% O_2 condition (see Fig. 16, page 50), this type of activity was not useful to get insight into the postulated limitations of mitochondrial function at 20% O_2. Therefore, we applied electrical stimulus trains (10 s, 20 Hz) as another experimental tool to trigger temporally defined neuronal activation and associated mitochondrial redox responses (NAD(P)H and FAD fluorescence transients) in area CA3. Such stimulus trains are well tolerated by hippocampal tissue (Schuchmann et al., 2001; Foster et al., 2005; Kann et al., 2005), and it was demonstrated that there are tight positive correlations between neuronal activation and redox responses over a wide range of stimulus intensities and frequencies (5, 20, 100 Hz) (Kann et al., 2003a).

4.3.1 Quantification of interstitial pO_2

We quantify interstitial pO_2 levels under both oxygenation conditions (20% O_2 and 95% O_2) and during electrical stimulation by using an O_2 sensor microelectrode. During the 95% O_2 condition we determined a pO_2 of 578±17 mmHg (n=9) at the surface of the slice (Fig. 8C). That was considerably lower compared to ACSF saturated with 95% O_2 at 24°C in the storage container (694 mmHg). The difference reflected a loss of ~15% of O_2 tension because of the diffusion from ACSF to the ambient atmosphere with an O_2 fraction of about 21%. This fact also explains why there was no discrepancy at 20% O_2. The measured pO_2 of 148±2 mmHg (n=9) closely matched the estimation for 24°C (146 mmHg). In a depth of 100 µm, the pO_2 was considerably lower (Fig. 8A, C), indicating substantial O_2 consumption as a result of metabolic demands of neurons and glial cells (Attwell and Iadecola, 2002; Thompson et al., 2003). When comparing the 95% and 20% O_2 conditions, the pO_2 in the slice core dropped

Results

from 472±11 to 51±4 mmHg (n=18) (Fig. 8A, C). This refers to hyperoxic and normoxic conditions, respectively, according to *in vivo* data (Rolett et al., 2000; Erecinska and Silver, 2001). During electrical stimulation, the pO_2 rapidly decreased (Fig. 8A, B), which reflects enhanced O_2 consumption of the mitochondrial ETC (Foster et al., 2005; Hayakawa et al., 2005). At 95% O_2 the lowest pO_2 was 293 mmHg and thus still clearly hyperoxic. At 20% O_2 the pO_2 decreased on average to 24.9±2 mmHg (n=18) (Fig. 8C, D) which is still in the normoxic range. Although electrical stimulation evoked nearly identical transient increases in $[K^+]_o$ under both oxygenation conditions, amplitudes of pO_2 transients (Fig. 8B, D) and integrals as determined from onset to nadir of pO_2 transients were significantly reduced at 20% O_2 (reduction to 63±8% as normalized to 95% O_2 condition, n=18, p<0.001). These observations might indicate a significant reduction in O_2 availability during stimulation in the 20% O_2 condition. The rise times of pO_2 transients during stimulation were not significantly different under both oxygenation conditions. In contrast, the decay time was significantly prolonged at 20% O_2 (Fig. 8E), which was suggestive for a reduced O_2 diffusion gradient from the surface to slice core.

These data indicate that during spontaneous network activities and electrically evoked neuronal activation, interstitial pO_2 values in the slice core were hyperoxic at 95% O_2 and, according to *in vivo* data (Rolett et al., 2000; Erecinska and Silver, 2001), in the normoxic range at 20% O_2.
We next explored the mitochondrial redox state during the 20% and 95% O_2 condition, and during neuronal activation evoked by electrical stimulation.

Results

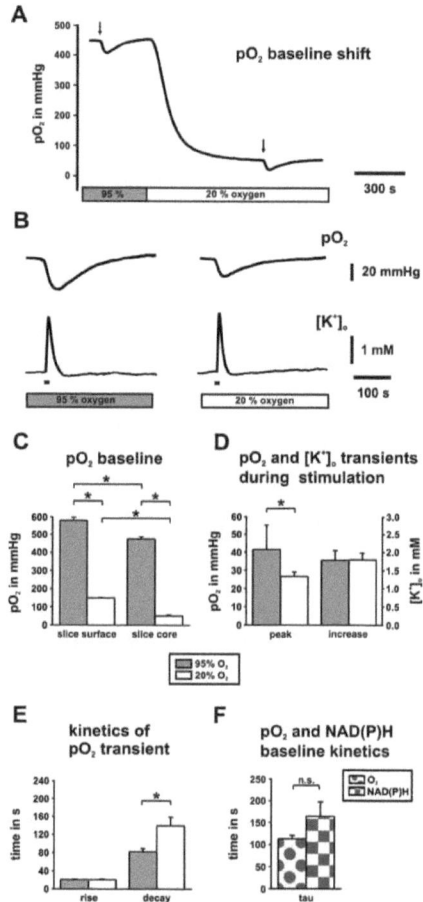

Figure 8. Absolute values of interstitial pO_2.

The O_2 sensor microelectrode was positioned in SP and the pO_2 was continuously measured. Note that "95% O_2" (grey bars) and "20% O_2" (white bars) refer to saturation levels of ACSF in the storage container. **(A)** The pO_2 baseline shift was measured in the slice core (100 μm depth). Each small pO_2 transient corresponds to enhanced O_2 consumption during neuronal activation evoked by electrical stimulation (10 s, 20 Hz, black arrows) to the fibre tracts from dentate gyrus to area CA3. **(B)** Traces on an expanded time scale illustrate that pO_2 transients were smaller at 20% O_2, although transient increases in $[K^+]_o$ were similar. **(C)** Histograms summarizing pO_2 baseline values which were determined at the surface and in the slice core. Note the significant smaller pO_2 values in the slice core under both oxygenation conditions. **(D)** pO_2 transients during electrical stimulation were significantly smaller at 20% O_2. Note that there is no difference in the amplitudes of $[K^+]_o$ transients, indicating virtually the same degree of neuronal activation under both O_2 conditions. **(E)** Rise and decay times of pO_2 transients during stimulation are given for the 10-90% interval. Note the significantly slower decay time at 20% O_2. **(F)** Kinetics of NAD(P)H and pO_2 baseline shifts are not significantly different, indicating a tight correlation between mitochondrial redox state and pO_2. Recordings were made in area CA3 of rat OHSCs under submerged conditions. *p<0.05

Results

4.3.2 Quantification of NAD(P)H and FAD fluorescence

Changes in the intensity of NAD(P)H and FAD fluorescence primarily reflect changes in mitochondrial redox state, in particular in brain slice preparations in which artefacts due to adaptations in blood flow are absent (Lipton, 1973; Kann et al., 2003a). We quantify changes in mitochondrial redox state during both oxygenation conditions by monitoring changes in NAD(P)H and FAD fluorescence.

Switching from 95% to 20% O_2 resulted in substantial elevation of NAD(P)H fluorescence baseline (8.8±1.9%, n=5) (Fig. 9A), which was reversible and indicated less oxidation of the dinucleotide pool by the mitochondrial ETC (Mayevsky and Chance, 1975; Foster et al., 2005). The time constant of NAD(P)H baseline elevation (163±27 s, n=5) and the time constant of the pO_2 decrease (112±7 s, n=4) were not significantly different (p=0.18) (Fig. 8F), suggesting a tight correlation between changes in mitochondrial redox state and pO_2 (Fig. 8A, 9A).

Next, we determined the mitochondrial redox state during 20% O_2 compared to 95% O_2 by monitoring stimulus-evoked NAD(P)H and FAD fluorescence transients in CA3 of rat OHSCs. NAD(P)H fluorescence transients showed the characteristic dip and overshoot components in both oxygenation conditions, whereas the amplitudes and kinetics of the biphasic transients differed markedly. At 20% O_2, the dip component indicating enhanced NAD(P)H oxygenation already terminated during stimulus trains of 10 s (Fig. 9A), which was also reflected by significantly shortened rise and decay times of the dip (Fig. 9B). Taking both time to peak of the dip component of the NAD(P)H transient and the data from interstitial pO_2 recordings at 20% O_2 (Fig. 8) into account, we estimated a threshold of 41±5 mmHg (n=18) in the slice core for a transient limitation of mitochondrial oxidation. The amplitude of the dip component did not differ under both oxygenation conditions when fluorescence was recorded from the whole CA3 area using photomultiplier-based microfluorimetry. However, by using CCD-camera based fluorescence recordings, which gives us the opportunity to distinguish between different layers of area CA3, the amplitude of the dip component was significantly reduced (from 1.25±0.09% to 0.79±0.09%, n=18, p=0.001) during the 20% O_2 condition compared to the 95% O_2 condition within stratum radiatum (where the stimulated fibre tracts terminate on the dendrites of CA3 neurons), indicating a higher degree of oxidative limitations in this region (Fig. 10B, C). At 95% O_2, the dip component was not unlimited because extended stimulus trains of 20, 30, 40 (data not shown), and 60 s at 10 Hz (Fig. 9A,

Results

lower trace) revealed a maximal time to the negative peak of 13.7±1 s (n=16). Taking into account that the increase in $[K^+]_o$ also reached a maximum after 13±2 s (n=6), this leads to the suggestion that it reflects a transient exhaustion of neurotransmission.

Amplitudes of the overshoot components of the NAD(P)H transients were significantly larger at 20% O_2 in both regions stratum radiatum and stratum pyramidale (Fig. 9B, 10B, 10C), whereas the effect was more prominent in stratum radiatum, which reaffirm the suggestion of higher O_2 sensitivity of the synaptic compartment. By monitoring the amplitudes (1.56±0.1 mM versus 1.47±0.2 mM, n=8, p=0.67) and the kinetics of $[K^+]_o$ transients during identical stimulus trains (Fig. 9A, C), it could be excluded that the difference in amplitudes and kinetics of the NAD(P)H transients were caused by less neuronal activation at 20% O_2.

FAD fluorescence, which is more specific for mitochondria (Scholz et al., 1969; Kunz and Kunz, 1985; Huang et al., 2002), was recorded simultaneously with changes in NAD(P)H fluorescence. Biphasic FAD transients were inverse in shape because of different fluorescence properties of flavin adenine dinucleotides (Shuttleworth et al., 2003; Kann and Kovács, 2007), and they consisted of a peak and a subsequent undershoot component. The effects of tissue oxygenation were also evident for stimulus-evoked FAD transients (Fig. 10B, D), and thus substantiated the finding of transient limitation of oxidation at 20% O_2 in mitochondria.

The tight correlation between changes in mitochondrial redox state and pO_2 was implied by overlaying traces of NAD(P)H and pO_2 transients under both oxygenation conditions (Fig. 10E) as well as by the fact that decay time constants of NAD(P)H overshoot and pO_2 transients were not significantly different (Fig. 10F).

The data indicate that mitochondrial redox state and pO_2 are tightly coupled and that electrical stimuli reveal transient alterations in redox responses when pO_2 decrease within the normoxic range. NAD(P)H and FAD fluorescence transients elicit limitation of mitochondrial oxidative capacity during 20% O_2. It was also demonstrated that evoked mitochondrial redox responses differ in somatic and synaptic neuronal compartments, which suggests that the synaptic compartment of area CA3 (stratum radiatum) is more sensitive to decreases in tissue pO_2 compared to the somatic compartment of area CA3 (stratum pyramidale).

Results

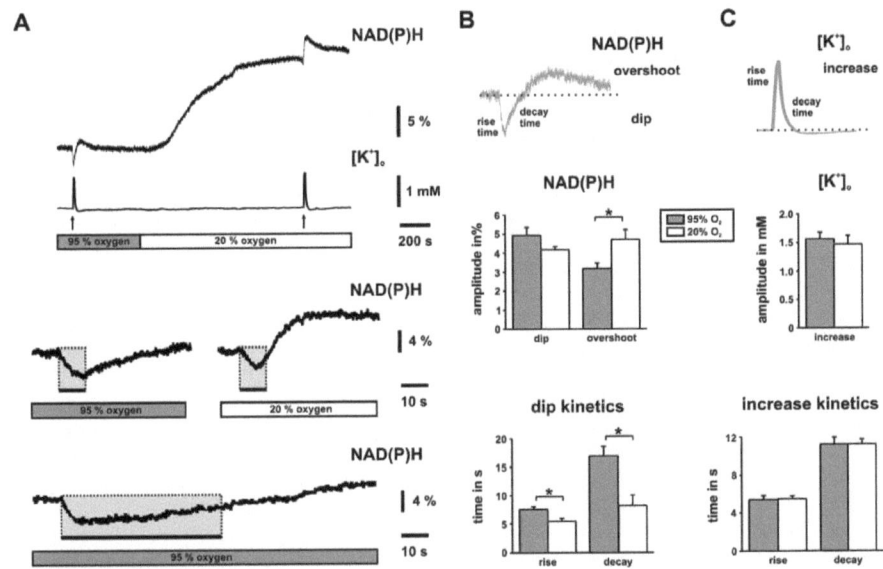

Figure 9. Changes in NAD(P)H fluorescence and $[K^+]_o$.
(A) The substantial NAD(P)H baseline elevation at 20% O_2 indicates reduced oxidation of the dinucleotide pools. Brief stimulus trains (10 s, 20 Hz, black arrows and bars) elicited biphasic NAD(P)H transients with different shapes under both oxygenation conditions (grey and white bars). The traces in the middle are from another experiment and displayed on an enlarged time scale. At 20% O_2, the biphasic NAD(P)H transient is characterized by a briefer initial dip component (grey rectangles) and a more rapidly developing and pronounced overshoot component. Note that the dip component terminates before the end of the stimulus train (right black bar). The bottom trace illustrates a NAD(P)H transient during a stimulus train of 60 s (20 Hz). (B) Pairs of stimulus-evoked biphasic NAD(P)H transients (n=8) were analyzed for amplitudes of dip (given as a positive value) and overshoot components as well as for dip kinetics (illustrated in scheme). Note that NAD(P)H originated as the sum of fluorescence from SP and SR and that $[K^+]_o$ was simultaneously recorded in SP to quantify neuronal activation.
(C) Pairs of stimulus-evoked transient increases in $[K^+]_o$ (n=8) were analyzed for amplitudes and kinetics (illustrated in scheme). Rise and decay times are given for 10-90% intervals. Recordings were made in area CA3 of rat OHSCs under submerged conditions. *$p<0.05$

Results

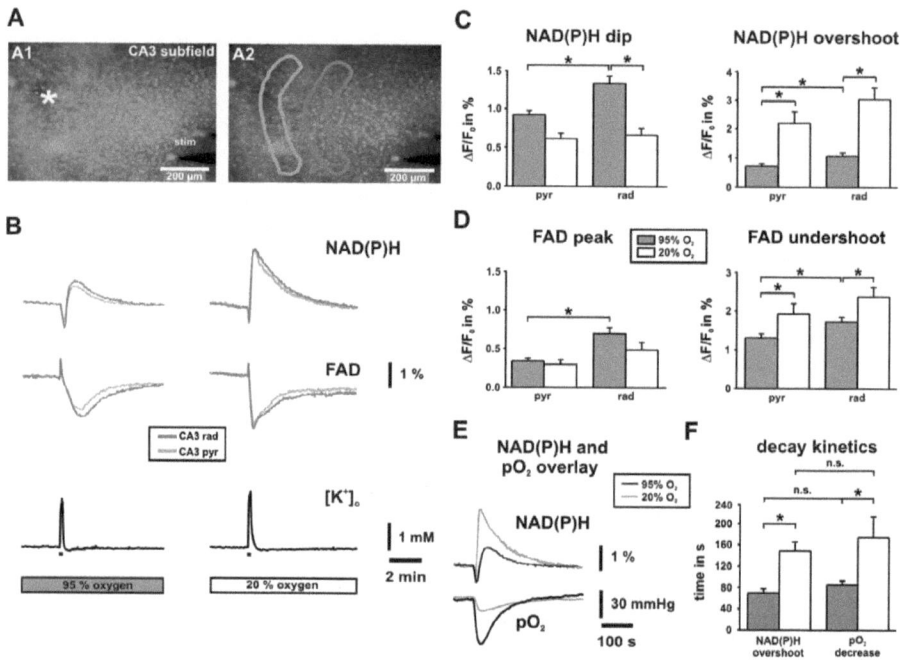

Figure 10. Stimulus-evoked NAD(P)H and FAD fluorescence transients in stratum pyramidale and stratum radiatum of area CA3.

(**A**) Overlay of NAD(P)H and FAD fluorescence images as recorded with a delay of 130 ms. The K$^+$-sensitive electrode was positioned in SP (white asterisk), the bipolar stimulation electrode close to the dentate gyrus (stim) for electrical activation of fibre tracts to CA3. ROIs (light grey, SP; dark grey, SR) were selected to determine changes in %ΔF/F$_0$ from image stacks that were recorded at 0.5 Hz. (**B**) The shapes of biphasic NAD(P)H (top traces) and FAD (middle traces) fluorescence transients as evoked by stimulus trains (10 s, 20 Hz, black bars) are clearly distinct at 20% O$_2$. Note that FAD transients (peak and undershoot) are inverse to NAD(P)H transients (dip and overshoot) because of different fluorescence properties of the dinucleotides. Transient increases in [K$^+$]$_o$ as evoked by stimulus trains were simultaneously recorded (bottom trace) and indicate virtually the same degree of neuronal activation at 95 and 20% O$_2$ (2.1±0.1 and 2.4±0.2 mM, n=18, p=0.26). (**C**)(**D**) Histograms summarizing the analysis of NAD(P)H and FAD transients (n=18 each) in SP (pyr) and SR (rad). Note that differences are most prominent in SR. (**E**) Overlay of NAD(P)H and pO$_2$ transients in SP as evoked by stimulus trains. (**F**) Histogram summarizing the decay time constant of NAD(P)H overshoots and pO$_2$ transients at 95% O$_2$ and 20% O$_2$ (n=18). Recordings were made in rat OHSCs under submerged conditions. *p<0.05

Results

4.4 O_2 consumption and mitochondrial redox state during gamma oscillations

The findings that gamma oscillations were highly sensitive to decreases in tissue pO_2 and NAD(P)H and pO_2 transients were altered at low tissue pO_2, led us to the hypothesis that this might have been mediated by limitations of mitochondrial function. To get further insight, we monitored the O_2 consumption during gamma oscillations and tested the effects of the specific complex I inhibitor rotenone. We compared different forms of evoked neuronal activity, namely neuronal activation as evoked by electrical stimulus trains (10 s, 20 Hz), gamma oscillations and low Mg^{2+}-induced epileptiform activity, and classified them according to their O_2 consumption. Finally, we monitored the mitochondrial redox state during gamma oscillations by recording stimulus-evoked NAD(P)H and FAD fluorescence transients to determine whether mitochondrial oxidative capacity is limited during gamma oscillations.

4.4.1 Interstitial pO_2 during spontaneous activity and during gamma oscillations in acute mouse hippocampal slices

O_2 consumption was determined by Clark-style O_2 sensor microelectrodes at various depths (40 μm to 160 μm below the cut slice surface) in acute mouse hippocampal slices during spontaneous neuronal network activity and, subsequently, during persistent gamma oscillations that were induced by ACh application and verified by local field potential recordings in each subfield (not shown, but see Fig. 4A). Depth profiles showed that pO_2 strongly decreased with depth in slices (Fig. 11A), indicating substantial O_2 consumption due to metabolic demand of active neurons and glial cells (Attwell and Iadecola, 2002). This effect was also observed in rat OHSCs (see Fig. 8A, C), where the tissue pO_2 of the slice core was significantly decreased compared to the tissue pO_2 of the slice surface. Overall, pO_2 was lower in area CA3 compared with area CA1 (Fig. 11B, lower left histogram) and dentate gyrus (not shown), presumably reflecting differences in spontaneous activity and concomitant metabolic activity. Importantly, during robust and persistent gamma oscillations (>30 min of onset), pO_2 was further decreased significantly in both CA3 and CA1 (Fig. 11B, upper histograms), indicating sustained additional increases in O_2 consumption. Calculating the decrease in pO_2 (in %) during gamma oscillations relative to pO_2 during spontaneous activity revealed that O_2 consumption was highest in CA3 (Fig. 11B, lower right histogram). This was consistent with observations that gamma oscillations were more prominent in area CA3 (Fig. 4; Fisahn et al., 1998). The fact that higher O_2 consumption in CA3 was only evident in a depth of 160 μm might be explained by the more intact network structure and thus network function in a greater distance from the cut slice surface.

These data suggest that gamma oscillations are associated with sustained high O_2 consumption and require proper mitochondrial oxidative metabolism.

Results

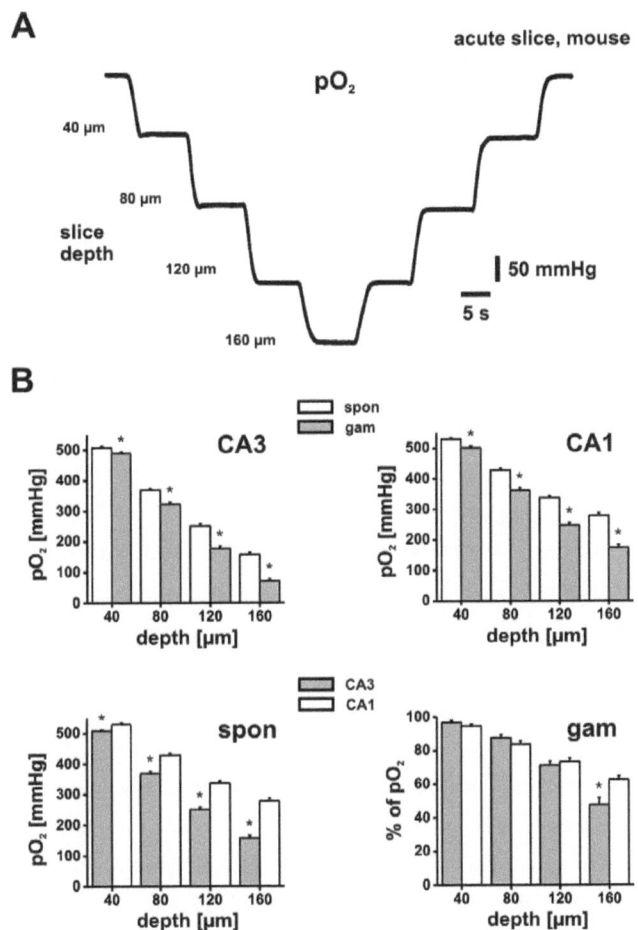

Figure 11. O₂ consumption during gamma oscillations in acute mouse hippocampal slices.

(A) Depth profiles of interstitial pO$_2$ ranging from 40 µm to 160 µm below the cut slice surface were determined in area CA3 (trace) and area CA1 using O$_2$ sensor microelectrodes. (B) Absolute values of pO$_2$ in a given slice were obtained during spontaneous network activity (spon) and subsequently during gamma oscillations (gam) that were evoked by bath application of ACh (2 µM) and physostigmine (400 nM). Note that robust and persistent gamma oscillations had been present for >30 min before depth profiles were made. The histograms summarize pO$_2$ values from multiple depth profiles (n>16) in eight slices. Note that the interstitial pO$_2$ decreases significantly during gamma oscillations in both CA3 and CA1 (upper histograms) while O$_2$ consumption during gamma oscillations is highest in CA3 (lower right). Recordings were made under interface conditions. *$p<0.05$

4.4.2 O$_2$ consumption during gamma oscillations in rat OHSCs

To test whether gamma oscillations in rat OHSCs also consume high amounts of O$_2$ we measured the absolute O$_2$ tension within the slice core of area CA3 (100 µm depth) during ACh application and during initial and persistent oscillatory activity. We recorded under submerged conditions, where application of ACh and physostigmine also resulted in robust and persistent gamma oscillations (Fig. 12). Application of ACh and physostigmine immediately led to a steep increase of O$_2$ consumption with a peak of 117.14±12.5 mmHg (n=7). After 1-2 min of sustained ACh application gamma oscillations with high amplitudes were observed (Fig. 12C, D). Ongoing and persistent gamma oscillations consumed continually high amounts of O$_2$, after 12 min of ACh application the O$_2$ consumption was still highly increased (82.86±13.4 mmHg, n=7), which supports our finding from acute slices that there is a considerable increase in O$_2$ consumption during gamma oscillations (Fig. 11). However, the O$_2$ consumption after 12 min of persistent gamma oscillations was significantly less increased in relation to the maximal peak of the pO$_2$ transient (p=0.005, n=7) (Fig. 12) and also the gamma power was significantly reduced. The Gaussian fit of the power spectrum showed a significant reduction of height and area under the curve (see Table 2).

During persistent gamma oscillations we applied rotenone, a specific and irreversible complex I inhibitor, to investigate the influence of mitochondria function on O$_2$ consumption. Continuous bath application of rotenone (1 µM), in presence of ACh and physostigmine promptly evoked a sustained pO$_2$ increase in CA3 (Fig. 12). The pO$_2$ gradually increased, whereas this effect was significant after 1 min of rotenone application (295.67±17.9 mmHg, n=7, p=0.02). Intriguingly, rotenone application was also associated with a significant loss in the power of gamma oscillations within the first 2 min (Fig. 12, Table 2). After 3 min of rotenone application the pO$_2$ does not significantly differ from baseline conditions (Fig. 12B, 318.33±18.9 mmHg versus 347.22±7.31 mmHg, p=0.14, n=7) and gamma oscillations were almost abolished (Fig. 12C, D, Table 2). In some experiments, we applied rotenone for up to 20 min, which resulted in a new steady-state of 83±9 mmHg (n=3) above baseline pO$_2$ prior to induction of gamma oscillations (not shown).

We also showed that application of 1 µM rotenone to OHSCs immediately led to a sustained increase in NAD(P)H autofluorescence in stratum pyramidale and stratum radiatum of area CA3 (Fig. 13), which reflects a decrease in mitochondrial oxidation and thus strengthened the suggestion that the fast decrease in gamma power during rotenone application depends on

Results

limitations in mitochondrial function. The inclination of the NAD(P)H signal from stratum pyramidale was significantly steeper in contrast to stratum radiatum, when comparing $\Delta F/F_o$ in % after 5, 10 and 20 min of rotenone application (p=0.04, p=0.04 and p=0.03, respectively, n=4, Fig. 13).

These data indicate that mitochondrial redox state is shifted to a more reduced state during rotenone application. This is supposed to lead to less ATP availability and thus to a decrease in gamma power. We note that rotenone did not result in spreading depolarization due to energy failure, which was in line with a previous report from acute hippocampal slices (Schuchmann et al., 2001). These data substantiate our evidence that gamma oscillations critically depend on mitochondrial oxidative energy metabolism and are highly sensitive to decreases in pO_2 (Huchzermeyer et al., 2008).

To estimate the degree of O_2 consumption during gamma oscillations more precisely, we next compare different forms of evoked neuronal activity; neuronal activation as evoked by electrical stimulus trains (10 s, 20 Hz), gamma oscillations and low Mg^{2+}-induced epileptiform activity and classify them with regard to their O_2 consumption.

Results

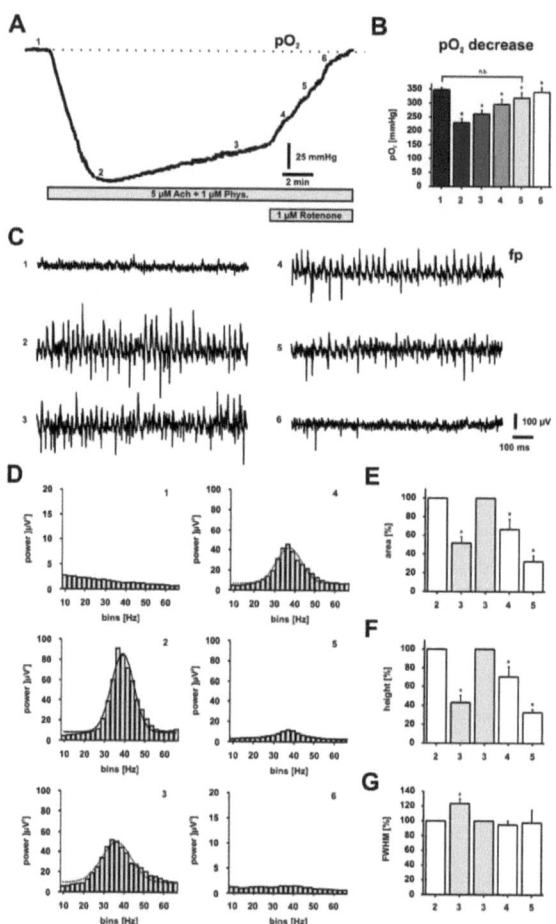

Figure 12. O_2 consumption and mitochondrial complex I inhibition in rat OHSCs.

(A) The interstitial pO_2 (trace) was monitored in the slice core (100 µm depth) of CA3 in rat OHSCs under submerged recording conditions. ACh and physostigmine were applied at concentrations of 5 µM and 1 µM, respectively. (B) Histogram summarizing absolute values of pO_2 during the six different conditions of the experiment (n=7). Note the significant increase in O_2 consumption during gamma oscillations (conditions 2 and 3) and its inhibition by bath application of the specific mitochondrial complex I inhibitor, rotenone (1 µM) (conditions 4 to 6). (C) Local field potential recordings were made in CA3 during the time course of the experiment as shown in A. Note that robust and persistent gamma oscillations (conditions 2 and 3) are completely blocked after 4-6 min of rotenone application (condition 6). (D) Power spectra were precisely approximated with a single Gaussian fit (see Results and Table 2). Area under the curve (E) and height (F) of Gaussian fit were significantly reduced after 11-13 min of ACh (condition 3, each with $p<0.001$, n=6), whereas FWHM was enhanced (G) ($p=0.013$, n=6), when data were normalized to condition 2. Moreover, area and height were significantly reduced during the first 2 min of rotenone application (condition 4, $p=0.029$ and $p=0.043$, n=6, respectively) and after 2-4 min of rotenone application (condition 5, each with $p<0.001$, n=6), when data were normalized to condition 3. *$p<0.05$

Results

	condition 2	condition 3	n	p-value
r^2	0.97 ± 0.01	0.96 ± 0.01	6	0.6
height	27.40 ± 10.6	12.28 ± 5.3	6	0.028 *
FWHM	10.49 ± 0.9	12.95 ± 1.3	6	0.028 *
width	8.92 ± 0.7	11 ± 1.1	6	0.028 *
area	335.16 ± 150	182.29 ± 85.5	6	0.028 *
	3	4		
r^2	0.96 ± 0.01	0.95 ± 0.01	6	0.735
height	12.28 ± 5.3	10.38 ± 5.2	6	0.028 *
FWHM	12.95 ± 1.3	12.25 ± 1.4	6	0.345
width	11 ± 1.1	10.40 ± 1.2	6	0.345
area	182.29 ± 85.5	145.97 ± 74.8	6	0.028 *
	3	5		
r^2	0.96 ± 0.01	0.93 ± 0.02	6	0.463
height	12.28 ± 5.3	3.46 ± 1.2	6	0.028 *
FWHM	12.95 ± 1.3	13.20 ± 3.3	6	0.917
width	11 ± 1.1	11.21 ± 2.8	6	0.917
area	182.29 ± 85.5	51.63 ± 18.3	6	0.028 *
	4	5		
r^2	0.95 ± 0.01	0.93 ± 0.02	6	0.917
height	10.38 ± 5.2	3.46 ± 1.2	6	0.028 *
FWHM	12.25 ± 1.4	13.20 ± 3.3	6	0.6
width	10.40 ± 1.2	11.21 ± 2.8	6	0.6
area	145.97 ± 74.8	51.63 ± 18.3	6	0.028 *

Table 2. Results from single Gaussian fits (Fig. 12D).
Abbreviations and units: correlation coefficient (r^2), full width at half maximum (**FWHM**; Hz), **area** ($\mu V^2 * Hz$) and **height** (μV^2). *p<0.05

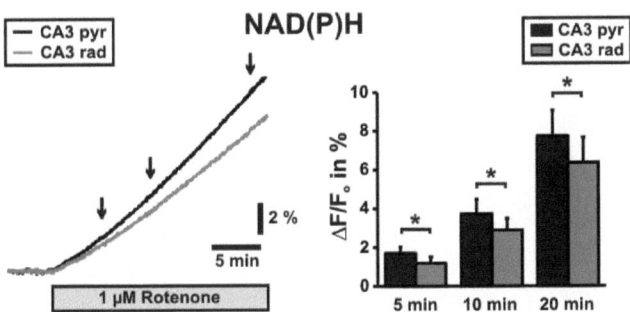

Figure 13. NAD(P)H fluorescence in stratum pyramidale and stratum radiatum of area CA3 during application of 1 µM rotenone.
Left: traces. Right: quantification of $\Delta F/F_o$ in % after 5, 10 and 20 min of rotenone application. Recordings were made in rat OHSCs under submerged conditions. *p<0.05

4.4.3 O_2 consumption of low Mg^{2+}-induced epileptiform activity

We investigated different forms of neuronal activity in area CA3 of rat OHSCs with respect to O_2 consumption. Therefore, we compared gamma oscillations with stimulus-evoked neuronal activation that elicit $[K^+]_o$ transients of <2 mM (Kann et al., 2003a) and with epileptiform activity that represent strong synchronized pathological neuronal activity (Kovács et al., 2001; 2005). Epileptiform activity, in the form of seizure-like events (SLEs) (Fig. 14), was induced by omitting Mg^{2+}-ions from the perfusion solution. This led to enhanced neuronal excitability due to removal of the voltage-dependent Mg^{2+} block from NMDA-activated channels as well as a decreased surface charge screening that results in facilitation of inward currents and transmitter release (Mody et al., 1987; Hamon et al., 1987)

Intriguingly, O_2 consumption during neuronal activation as evoked by electrical stimulation trains was considerably lower (42.7±6 mmHg, n=9) (Fig. 15) compared with gamma oscillations (86.11±10.67 mmHg, n=9) (Fig. 12A, B, 15C). In contrast, SLEs were accompanied by a massive increase in O_2 consumption with a maximum of 107±8 mmHg (n=9), similar to gamma oscillations (Fig. 14, 15, 12A, B, 15C). SLEs occured with an onset of 11.3±1.8 min (n=9) and elicited pO_2 transients with a duration of 5.28±0.4 min (n=9).

These data suggest that gamma oscillations represent neuronal network activity of high degree and are associated with high O_2 consumption due to enhanced oxidative energy metabolism.

To test whether the high degree of O_2 consumption during gamma oscillations leads to a limitation in mitochondrial oxidative capacity, we next explored mitochondrial redox state during gamma oscillations by applying NAD(P)H and FAD fluorescence imaging.

Results

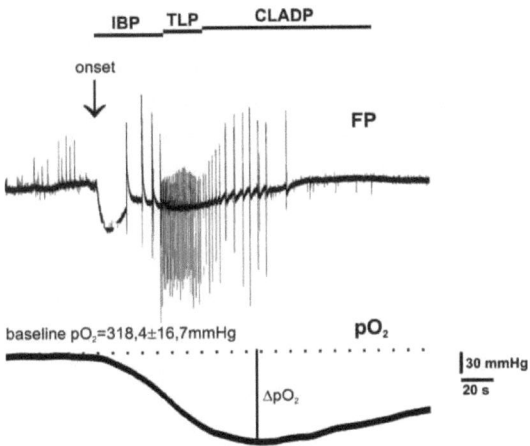

Figure 14. O_2 consumption during low Mg^{2+}-induced epileptiform activity.
Local field potential and pO_2 were recorded in SP. Epileptiform activity was induced by omitting Mg^{2+} ions from the recording solution and was characterized by an initial bursting period (IBP), followed by a tonic like period (TLP) and a longer clonic-like after discharge period (CLADP). Recordings were made in area CA3 of rat OHSCs under submerged conditions.

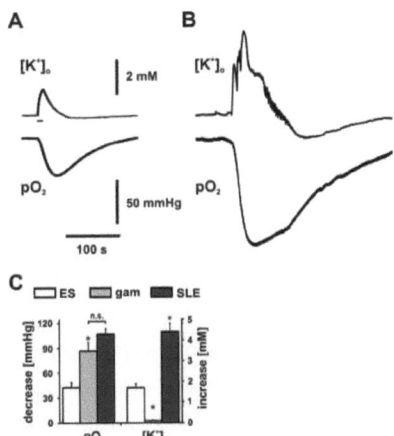

Figure 15. O_2 and $[K^+]_o$ transients during different types of neuronal activity.
(A) O_2 and $[K^+]_o$ transients of neuronal activation as evoked by electrical stimulation trains (20 Hz, 10 s) and **(B)** SLEs. **(C)** Histogram summarizing decreases in pO_2 (left) and increases in $[K^+]_o$ (right) during electrical stimulation (ES, 10 s, 20 Hz, n=9), gamma oscillations (gam, for pO_2 see Fig. 12A, B, condition 3, for $[K^+]_o$ see Fig. 16A, n =9) and SLEs (n=9). Recordings were made in area CA3 of rat OHSCs under submerged conditions. *$p<0.05$

4.4.4 Mitochondrial redox state during gamma oscillations

Cholinerigic gamma oscillations in rat OHSCs are associated with an initial biphasic NAD(P)H transient that was followed by a long-lasting NAD(P)H fluorescence elevation when persistent gamma oscillations were present (Fig. 16A). The long-lasting NAD(P)H elevations were significantly larger in stratum radiatum compared to stratum pyramidale (1.87±0.1% versus 1.26±0.1%, n=8, p<0.001), demonstrating that evoked mitochondrial redox responses differ in somatic and synaptic neuronal compartments. In these experiments, ACh application initially evoked increases in $[K^+]_o$ with a peak of 0.39±0.05 mM, which was associated with a biphasic NAD(P)H transient, and a steady-state $[K^+]_o$ level of 0.06±0.02 mM after >15 min (n=8). The low steady-state level of $[K^+]_o$ during ongoing gamma oscillations presumably reflects an optimal distribution of synchronized neuronal activity in the network and effective localized K^+-uptake by glial cells. The initial $[K^+]_o$ transient that *per se* enhances neuronal excitability and promotes the induction of gamma oscillations (LeBeau et al., 2002) very likely explains our observation of a slight decrease in both power of gamma oscillations and O_2 consumption during the first 10 to 12 min of ACh application (Fig. 12). Long-lasting NAD(P)H elevations emerged slowly when persistent gamma oscillations were fully established at 118±12 s (n=8) after start of ACh application and on top of the initial biphasic NAD(P)H transient (Fig. 16A, black arrow). Interestingly, this experiment showed that gamma oscillations caused more reduction of nicotinamide adenine dinucleotide pool despite hyperoxic pO_2 levels, which might reflect stimulation of TCA cycle activity and/or attenuation of ETC activity.

To get further insight in the underlying mechanisms, we additionally applied electrical stimulation to evoke biphasic NAD(P)H and FAD fluorescence transients (Shuttleworth et al., 2003; Huchzermeyer et al., 2008). In the absence of gamma oscillations, characteristic biphasic NAD(P)H and FAD fluorescence transients were observed (Fig. 16C), clearly indicating that mitochondrial oxidation can be further increased by electrical stimulation in CA3. In the presence of gamma oscillations (>15 min of onset), components of electrical stimulus-evoked NAD(P)H and FAD fluorescence transients differed markedly. Most importantly, the peak component of FAD fluorescence transients was absent and the dip component of NAD(P)H fluorescence transients was significantly smaller in amplitude and showed faster kinetics (Fig. 16C), suggesting that the mitochondrial oxidative capacity was already utilized near limit during gamma oscillations. The observation that electrical

Results

stimulus-evoked NAD(P)H fluorescence transients showed weaker alterations than FAD fluorescence transients might be explained by the fact that FAD fluorescence is more specific for mitochondria (Kunz and Kunz, 1985; Huang et al., 2002). Indeed, applying confocal laser scanning microscopy in CA3 clearly demonstrated that NAD(P)H fluorescence originated from both mitochondria and cytosol while staining with potentiometric dye, rhodamine-123 was primarily mitochondrial (Fig. 16B; Kovács et al., 2005). Amplitudes of electrical stimulus-evoked $[K^+]_o$ transients did not differ in the absence and presence of gamma oscillations (Fig. 16C), indicating the same degree of enhanced neuronal activity. Nevertheless, the decay time of $[K^+]_o$ transients as evoked during gamma oscillations was significantly prolonged, which might reflect limitations of Na^+/K^+-ATPase activity and/or glial K^+-buffering (Newman et al., 1984; D'Ambrosio et al., 2002). These data suggest that gamma oscillations are associated with utilization of mitochondrial oxidative capacity near limit and it was shown that NAD(P)H and FAD fluorescence transients are not implicitly coupled.

Results

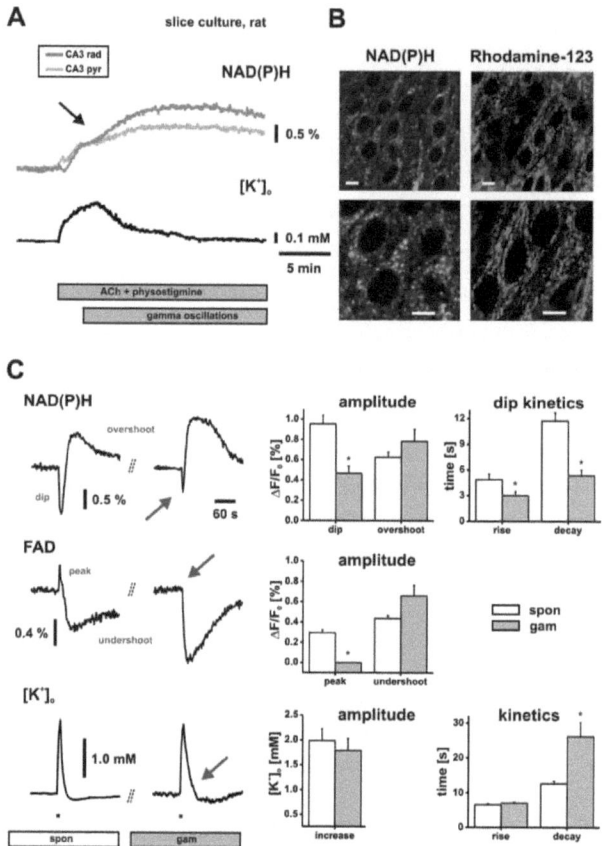

Figure 16. Mitochondrial redox state during gamma oscillations.
(A) Simultaneous recordings of NAD(P)H fluorescence in SP (light grey) and SR (dark grey) as well as $[K^+]_o$ and local field potentials (data not shown) in SP of area CA3 were made during application of ACh (10 μM, bottom grey bar). Initially, the increase in $[K^+]_o$ was associated with a biphasic NAD(P)H fluorescence transient (dip and overshoot component), which transformed into a persistent NAD(P)H elevation (black arrow) when gamma oscillations were fully established (illustrated as top grey bar). Note that persistent NAD(P)H elevation during gamma oscillations were significantly larger in SR. **(B)** Images as obtained by confocal laser scanning microscopy in SP of CA3. Note that NAD(P)H fluorescence originated from both mitochondria and cytosol (left) while rhodamine-123 staining was primarily mitochondrial (right). Neuronal nuclei showed the weakest fluorescence intensities. Scale bars denote 20 μm. **(C)** Simultaneous recordings of biphasic NAD(P)H and FAD fluorescence transients as well as of $[K^+]_o$ transients as evoked by electrical stimulation (10 s, 20 Hz, black spots) during spontaneous activity (spon) and in the presence of persistent gamma oscillations (gam) in area CA3. Note that during gamma oscillations amplitudes and kinetics of both NAD(P)H dip and FAD peak were clearly altered (red arrows, histograms). Note that the decay time of $[K^+]_o$ transients was significantly prolonged (red arrow) during gamma oscillations while the amplitude was unaffected (histograms). Rise and decay times were given for the 10-90% intervals. Histograms summarize data from different OHSCs (n=7). Recordings were made in rat OHSCs under submerged conditions. *p<0.05

4.5 Chronic rotenone model

Rotenone is a specific complex I inhibitor of the mitochondrial ETC. The finding that acute rotenone application (1 µM) abolished gamma oscillations and concomitant O_2 consumption (see Fig. 12) showed that gamma oscillations critically depend on mitochondrial oxidative energy metabolism. Moreover, we showed that the NAD(P)H redox state during acute rotenone application was shifted to a more reduced state which clearly demonstrate that mitochondrial redox state is altered during acute rotenone application.
From other studies it is known that rotenone concentrations between 1 µM (Schuchmann et al., 2001) and 20 µM (Gerich et al., 2006) in slice preparations show strong effects in acute experiments.
We tested whether also chronic inhibition of complex I with rotenone might lead to alterations in functional performances of mitochondria. Therefore, we established an *in vitro* model where low concentrations of rotenone were applied for several days (chronic rotenone model).

4.5.1 Chronic rotenone application and neuronal cell death

We treated rat OHSCs from day 3 to day 8 after preparation with 10, 20 and 50 nM rotenone, respectively, to determine appropriate rotenone concentrations and the duration of the chronic application. As 100% positive controls slice cultures were incubated with 5 µM NMDA and 5 µM KA for 24 hours before they were fixated.
We quantified the amount of degenerated neurons within the cell layers of CA3, CA1 and dentate gyrus (Fig. 17) by using FJB as a fluorescent marker. The quantification showed that there were no significant differences between the amounts of FJB-positive cells in the slice cultures treated with 10 or 20 nM rotenone compared to controls (Fig. 17A, B). Slice cultures which were treated with 50 nM rotenone for 5 *div* showed a complete disruption of the tissue and thus were taken out from evaluation. Conversely, application of NMDA and KA for 24 hours resulted in an almost complete cell death in all regions (Fig. 17 A, B).

Results

4.5.2 Mitochondrial redox responses during chronic rotenone application

For the *in vitro* model we determined the lowest concentration of rotenone (10 nM) which did not cause enhanced neuronal cell death. We tested whether the mitochondrial redox state in these OHSCs was altered in relation to control slices (Fig. 18). Therefore, we induced neuronal activation in area CA3 by electrical stimulation which led to an increase in $[K^+]_o$ which was not significantly different compared to the $[K^+]_o$ increase in control slices (1.84±0.2 mM, n=8 and 2.16±0.2 mM, n=15 respectively, p=0.32) (Fig. 18 A, B). Interestingly, associated FAD transients in rotenone-treated OHSCs showed a significant reduction in peak amplitude (0.74±0.1%, n=8 versus 0.10±0.01%, n=15, p<0.001), although amplitudes of NAD(P)H dips were not significantly different compared to control slices (0.93±0.1%, n=8 versus 1.08±0.2%, n=15, p=0.38) (Fig. 18 A, B).

These data indicate that chronic application of low concentrations of the complex I inhibitor rotenone does not lead to enhanced cell death in OHSCs but to altered mitochondrial redox responses which are similar but not equal to the alterations of biphasic redox transients observed during gamma oscillations. Moreover, these data support the finding that NAD(P)H and FAD fluorescence transients are not implicitly coupled.

Results

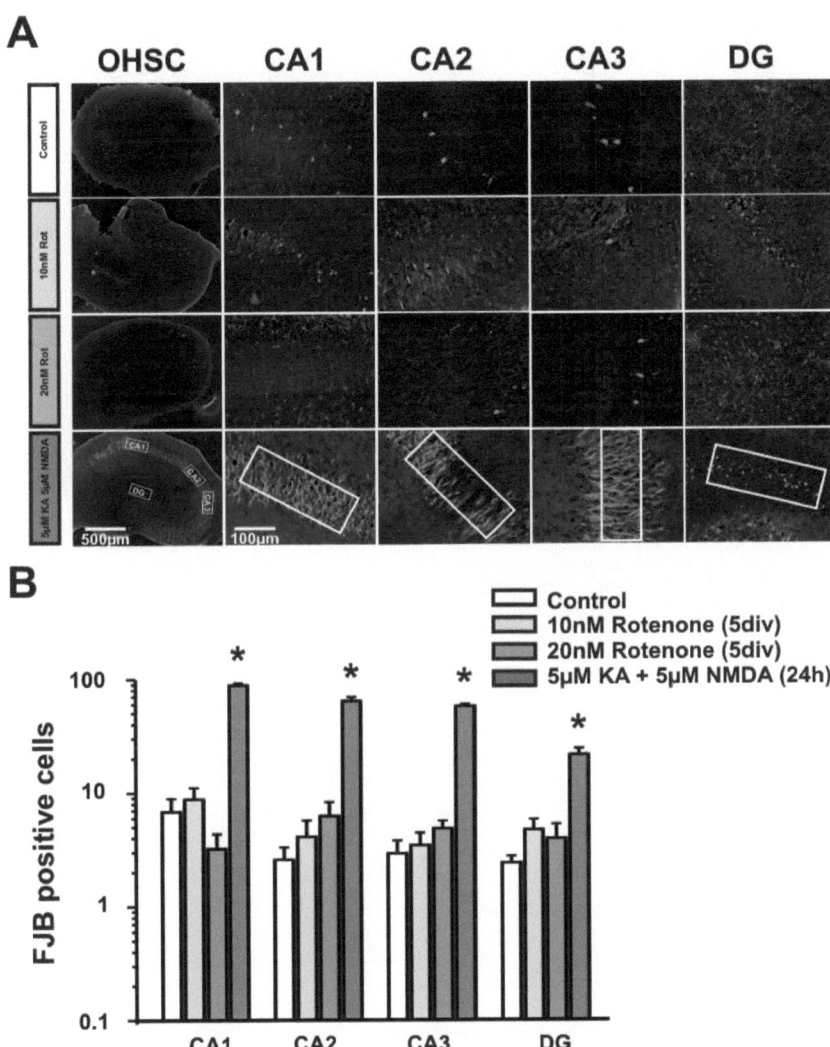

Figure 17. Quantification of neuronal cell death after chronic rotenone application.
(A) FJB staining of rat OHSCs treated with 10 nM or 20 nM rotenone or 5 µM KA and 5 µM NMDA, respectively. White squares indicate ROIs, in which the amount of FJB-positve cells was quantified. (B) Evaluation of FJB-positve cells. Data from 7 animals were averaged for each of the following conditions: control (n=21), 10 nM rotenone for 5 *div* (n=16), 20 nM rotenone for 5 *div* (n=14) and 5 µM KA and 5 µM NMDA for 24 h (n=16). Note that there were no significant differences between rotenone-treated OHSCs and control slices. *$p<0.05$

Results

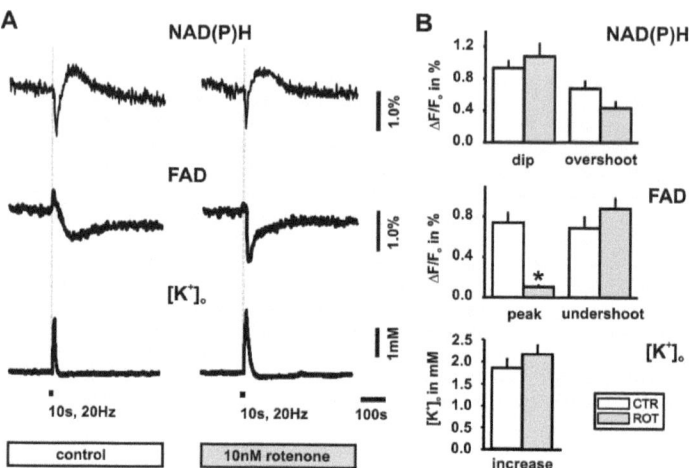

Figure 18. Mitochondrial redox responses during chronic rotenone application.

(A) Brief stimulus trains (10 s, 20 Hz, black bars) elicit NAD(P)H and FAD fluorescence transients with significantly reduced FAD peak amplitudes in rotenone (10 nM) -treated OHSCs compared to control slices. Note that the $[K^+]_o$ increases during stimuli were not significantly different. (B) Quantification of traces in A. Recordings were made in area CA3 under submerged conditions. *p<0.05

5 Discussion

This study addressed the O_2 and energy demands of gamma oscillations in area CA3 of hippocampal slice preparations.

In the first part it was shown that gamma oscillation in hippocampal slice preparations can be induced by ACh and that **(1)** cholinergic gamma oscillations have similar properties in acute mouse hippocampal slices and in rat OHSCs.

Further, we investigated the sensitivity of gamma oscillations to decreases in tissue pO_2 in relation to other forms of neuronal activity. We show that **(2)** gamma oscillations and spontaneous network activity decrease significantly at pO_2 levels that do not affect neuronal population responses as elicited by electrical stimuli, **(3)** pO_2 and mitochondrial redox state are tightly coupled, **(4)** electrical stimuli reveal transient alterations of redox responses when pO_2 decreases within the normoxic range, and **(5)** redox responses as evoked in somatic and synaptic neuronal compartments show different sensitivity to changes in pO_2.

In the next part we determined the O_2 demands of gamma oscillations. Therefore, we compared different forms of neuronal activity with regard to concomitant O_2 consumption. We further addressed the question whether O_2 consumption during gamma oscillations is dependent on proper mitochondrial function by applying the complex I inhibitor rotenone. The main findings are **(6)** robust and persistent gamma oscillations are associated with high levels of O_2 consumption, **(7)** these findings are most prominent in area CA3, **(8)** gamma oscillations of high power require utilization of mitochondrial oxidative capacity near limit, and **(9)** gamma oscillations are very sensitive to complex I inhibition.

We established an *in vitro* model for complex I inhibition to test the effects of chronic rotenone application. It is demonstrated that **(10)** chronic rotenone treatment in the nanomolar range does not lead to enhanced cell death but to **(11)** altered mitochondrial redox responses which are similar to mitochondrial redox responses that are evoked during gamma oscillations.

Discussion

Our data show that gamma oscillations are highly sensitive to decreases in tissue pO_2 and are associated with enhanced utilization of mitochondrial oxidative metabolism. We have demonstrated that O_2 consumption during gamma oscillations is highly increased and that complex I inhibition with rotenone leads to dramatic decreases in the gamma power.

This leads to the suggestion that gamma oscillations are associated with high energy consumption and require outstanding functional performance of neuronal mitochondria.

5.1 Gamma oscillations and their sensitivity to changes in pO_2

We investigated cholinergic gamma oscillations in rat OHSCs and acute mouse hippocampal slices under submerged and interface recording conditions. We have shown that gamma oscillations are more prominent in area CA3 compared to area CA1 in both kind of slice preparations and in both recording conditions. Similar findings have been reported in acute rat hippocampal slices (Fisahn et al., 1998) and *in vivo* (Bragin et al., 1995) which leads to the suggestion that this is a common feature for rodent hippocampal gamma oscillations.

Furthermore, gamma oscillations in area CA1 are characterized by a phase lag of >1 ms in both preparations, indicating neuronal network propagation from CA3 (Fisahn et al., 1998) where the gamma oscillations are supposed to be generated. The fact that gamma oscillations are generated in the CA3 area is strengthened by the observation of an intrinsic network oscillator in the hippocampal subregion (Fischer, 2003). Not only neuronal network oscillations in the gamma frequency range but also sharp wave-ripple oscillations have been reported to propagate in hippocampal slices in the millisecond time scale (Whittington et al., 1997; Fuchs et al., 2001; Both et al., 2008).

We have shown that gamma oscillations and also spontaneous network activity are highly sensitive to decreases in pO_2 within the range from ~450 mmHg (95% O_2) to ~50 mmHg (20% O_2), whereas evoked neuronal population responses are more resistant. During cholinergic gamma oscillations, network synchronization is determined by fast AMPA (α-amino-3-hydroxy-5-methyl-4-isoxazolepropionic acid) receptor-mediated excitation and by fast $GABA_A$ receptor-mediated inhibition (Fisahn et al., 1998; Mann et al., 2005; Bartos et al., 2007). Thereby pyramidal cells generate action potentials in the range of 1-3 Hz, whereas certain interneurons fire action-potentials phase locked to each gamma cycle up to 40 Hz (Bragin et al., 1995; Hájos et al., 2004) and thus are thought to synchronize the network.

Discussion

Interestingly, several subtypes of GABAergic interneurons like parvalbumin (PV)-containing basket and axo-axonic cells express high levels of cytochrome c (CC), suggesting high metabolic rates (Gulyás et al., 2006). Not only the CC signal intensity has been shown to be stronger in GABAergic neurons but the number of mitochondria is also higher compared to pyramidal cells which have low firing rates and accordingly low levels of CC (Gulyás et al., 2006). Remarkably, it has been reported that the PV-containing interneurons have the highest activity level during gamma oscillations and also during almost all behaviour-associated hippocampal activity patterns (Klausberger et al., 2003). This strengthens our hypothesis that gamma oscillations strongly depend on proper mitochondrial function and thus on ATP availability and neurotransmitter formation to maintain both excitability and fast inhibition. Here one can speculate that subtle decreases in O_2 availability lead to suppressed mitochondrial function and consequently disturb the precise interplay of slow excitatory pyramidal cells and fast inhibitory interneurons during gamma oscillations. This suggestion is supported by the finding that fast spiking and slow spiking neurons during spontaneous network activity are both sensitive to decreases in pO_2. This indicates that a balance between excitation and inhibition exists, which could explain the fact that we neither observe pathological activity nor abnormal neuronal population responses during our recordings. However, because of the significant contribution of fast inhibition to the generation of gamma oscillations, fast-spiking interneurons might be a critical target for alterations in pO_2 and mitochondrial function (Ackermann et al., 1984; Fuchs et al., 2007; Hájos et al., 2009).

We have to emphasise that spontaneous network activity and gamma oscillations are already decreased at ~50 mmHg which is still in the normoxic range and in the upper range of values (15-60 mmHg) which have been observed in air-respiring rodents (Feng et al., 1988; Rolett et al., 2000; Erecinska and Silver, 2001; Takano et al., 2007), and the 'critical' pO_2 for a breakdown of steady-state aerobic metabolism has been reported between 7 and 9 mmHg (Rolett et al., 2000). However, it is difficult to compare our data with these studies because the *in vivo* recordings were made mainly in the cerebral cortex, partially with different techniques and notably in the presence of anaesthetics that can significantly interfere with both network oscillations and mitochondrial function (Whittington et al., 2000; Muravchick and Levy, 2006).

The high sensitivity of gamma oscillations to changes in pO_2 is possibly due to an increased conductance of local ATP-dependent K^+ channels (Fujimura et al., 1997). This could lead to a hyperpolarization of the neuron from a critical membrane potential which protects the neuron

Discussion

from uncontrolled firing and reduces the energy requirements (Fujimura et al., 1997; Yamada et al., 2001).
Other explanations for the high sensitivity of gamma oscillations to decreases in tissue pO_2 could be an amplification of activity-dependent neuronal acidification as a result of lactate production (Stenkamp et al., 2001) and/or alterations of glutamate/GABA metabolism and vesicle mobilization (Waagepetersen et al., 1999; Verstreken et al., 2005).
It is important to stress that such abnormal processes might particularly occur in presynaptic and postsynaptic structures with high ion fluxes and high energy demand, which critically rely on proper mitochondrial function and O_2 supply (Attwell and Iadecola, 2002).

5.2 O_2 consumption during gamma oscillations

We have shown that gamma oscillations are accompanied by substantial decreases in pO_2 in both acute mouse hippocampal slices and rat OHSCs. This suggests that gamma oscillations are highly energy consuming.
The gamma power is higher in area CA3 compared to area CA1. Accordingly, we also find higher pO_2 decreases during gamma oscillations in CA3 compared to CA1 indicating a tight correlation between mitochondrial O_2 consumption and the strength of neuronal network oscillations. However, sustained and rapid pO_2 decreases indicate enhanced mitochondrial O_2 consumption during gamma oscillations in both hippocampal subfields.
By comparing the O_2 consumption during different forms of neuronal activity, we have found that O_2 consumption during gamma oscillations is as high as O_2 consumption during low Mg^{2+}-induced epileptiform activity. From these data we conclude that O_2 consumption during gamma oscillations is of high degree. In accordance with this finding, we have shown that the mitochondrial oxidative capacity is already utilized near limit during gamma oscillations, since the dip component of the NAD(P)H fluorescent transients is significantly reduced and the peak component of the FAD fluorescent transient is even abolished. An *in vivo* study supports our finding of increased O_2 and thus energy demand during gamma oscillations by showing a tight correlation between hemodynamic signals and synchronized gamma oscillations (Niessing et al., 2005).

Discussion

5.3 O$_2$ availability in hippocampal slice preparations

The O$_2$ diffusion distance in slice preparations is about ~90-200 µm from the slice surface to the slice core and thus greater compared with ~25 µm from capillaries to neurons *in vivo* (Tata and Anderson, 2002; Turner et al., 2007). To allow appropriate oxygenation within the slice core one can increase the pO$_2$ in the perfusion solution and/or diminish the thickness of the slice. Acute slices contain non-vital superficial layers that are damaged by the cutting procedure which in turn might influence the O$_2$ supply of deeper layers while functioning as a barrier for O$_2$ (Lipinski, 1989; Gjedde, 2002; Gjedde et al., 2002). Therefore, we used OHSCs which have vital superficial layers to examine the O$_2$ availability during neuronal activation as evoked by electrical stimulus trains. OHSCs are half as thick as acute slices (~180 versus ~400 µm). This is beneficial because of the reduced diffusion distance for O$_2$, ions and drugs. We have shown that the neuronal activation is associated with rapid decreases in pO$_2$ and thus enhanced mitochondrial O$_2$ consumption. We use these O$_2$ transients as a tool to examine the O$_2$ availability during neuronal activation in the physiological range under two different oxygenation conditions (during 95% O$_2$, which is a hyperoxic condition and during 20% O$_2$, where spontaneous network activity and gamma oscillations are significantly decreased). O$_2$ transients are reduced and less variable under the 20% O$_2$ condition compared to the 95% O$_2$ condition which indicate a reduction in O$_2$ availability although the pO$_2$ is still in the normoxic range (24.9±2 mmHg). However, this value could be even lower in neuronal microdomains with high metabolic turnover. This assumption is supported by the finding that associated stimulus-evoked redox responses show stronger alterations in the synaptic compartment (see below). Mitochondria in neurons are typically heterogeneously distributed; with a higher density in regions proximal to sites of high ATP utilization and they also vary in number, size and enzyme activity (Wong-Riley, 1989; Waagepetersen et al., 1999; Popov et al., 2005). Consistent with our finding that redox responses show stronger alterations in the synaptic compartment, it was reported that the local ATP demand leads to clusters of mitochondria which are associated with synapses, both in the presynaptic compartments and in postsynaptic terminals (Jones, 1986). Based on this fact it is likely that synapses are more vulnerable to pO$_2$ decreases than other neuronal compartments. Moreover, it is suggested that clustering of mitochondria may account for steep intracellular O$_2$ gradients (Jones, 1986) and it was shown that the heterogeneous mitochondrial distribution leads to heterogeneous subcellular ATP supply during low O$_2$ conditions. Both the intracellular O$_2$ gradient and the

Discussion

heterogeneous subcellular ATP supply lead to the assumption that enzymes with a greater average distance to mitochondria (e.g. Na^+/K^+-ATPases) experience a more dramatic decrease in ATP concentration than enzymes in close proximity to mitochondria do (e.g. cytoplasmic enzymes) during low pO_2 conditions (Jones, 1986). This could explain why gamma oscillations which likely require enhanced Na^+/K^+-ATPases activity are dramatically reduced during low pO_2. This is supported by our finding that the decay time of stimulus-evoked potassium transients during gamma oscillations is significantly prolonged, which might reflect limitations of the Na^+/K^+-ATPase activity.

O_2 transients during the 95% O_2 condition show higher amplitudes and more variability compared to the 20% O_2 condition which could be explained by a reduced efficacy of O_2 consumption because of respiratory uncoupling (Andrews et al., 2005). The slow recovery of O_2 transients, particular during low pO_2, reflects the greater diffusion distances in slice preparations compared with the *in vivo* situation. Additionally, a reduced O_2 gradient from the slice surface to the slice core has to be considered at 20% O_2 (Tata and Anderson, 2002; Turner et al., 2007). Proper mitochondrial function relies on a steep gradient of O_2 to overcome its low diffusion velocity. Thus, one can speculate that a decreased diffusion velocity during 20% O_2 leads to transient local hypoxia in areas with high density of respiring mitochondria and/or during neuronal activity which is associated with high amounts of O_2 consumption. However, the low diffusion velocity of O_2 explains the dramatic pO_2 decreases in depth profiles in living hippocampal slices (see Fig. 11; Foster et al., 2005).

In vivo stimulus-evoked decreases in pO_2 as observed in our slice preparations occur only under exceptional conditions, i.e. during cortical spreading depression (Takano et al., 2007) that is associated with vasoconstriction in mice (Ayata et al., 2004), during electrical stimulation in the cerebellum, and when adaptations in blood flow are blocked (Offenhauser et al., 2005). Neuronal activation *in vivo* under physiological conditions is associated with biphasic changes in pO_2, an initial 'dip' component, reflecting activity-dependent O_2 consumption, and a subsequent 'overshoot' component due to a rise in cerebral blood flow and thus an increase in O_2 availability. Therefore, it is difficult to precisely relate our data from slice preparations to the *in vivo* situation.

Nevertheless, decreases in pO_2 during sustained gamma oscillations in OHSCs were more than 2-fold of those recorded during neuronal activation in the physiological range (Heinemann et al., 1990; Kann et al., 2003a) and did not differ from those recorded during

Discussion

SLEs. Based on these relations, we propose that O_2 consumption during gamma oscillations is of high degree.

Furthermore, our data suggest that there might be local hypoxia in slices under low pO_2 conditions. Based on our results we would propose to supply slice preparations with hyperoxic pO_2 to examine high frequency oscillations. The finding that proper O_2 supply is essential during sustained network activity is supported by a recent study which shows that the local O_2 level is critical for generation and propagation of spontaneously occurring sharp wave-ripple oscillations and cholinergic oscillations (Hájos et al., 2009).

5.4 Mitochondrial redox state as a marker for functional performance of mitochondria

We have demonstrated that the mitochondrial redox state and pO_2 are tightly coupled over a wide range of tissue oxygenation levels. During 95% O_2 condition (~450 mmHg), nicotinamide adenine and flavin adenine dinucleotide pools might have been overly oxidized (Mayevsky and Chance, 2007). Nevertheless, prominent initial dips of NAD(P)H transients and peaks of FAD transients during electrical stimulation reveal a high oxidative capacity in the tissue at hyperoxic pO_2. Moreover, stimulus-evoked NAD(P)H transients at 95% O_2 are similar to those observed *in vivo*, where sustained neuronal activation is associated with large NAD(P)H dips (Jöbsis et al., 1971; Mayevsky and Chance, 1975; LaManna et al., 1984), indicating that O_2 supply to the brain parenchyma is rapidly increased and allows enhanced mitochondrial electron transfer. In contrast, lowering interstitial pO_2 to ~50 mmHg (20% O_2 condition) markedly elevates NAD(P)H fluorescence and is associated with alterations of stimulus-evoked redox responses. Interestingly, similar but more pronounced alterations of evoked NAD(P)H transients were reported under hypoxic conditions *in vivo* (LaManna et al., 1984). This observation might lead to the conclusion that there is a reduced oxidative capacity of the mitochondrial ETC at 20% O_2, which also hinting at a transient limitation of complex mitochondrial functions like ATP production, Ca^{2+} handling and neurotransmitter formation (Waagepetersen et al., 1999; Kann and Kovács, 2007).

In accordance with the discussion of pO_2 levels, a reduced mitochondrial oxidative capacity might particular occur in neuronal microdomains with high metabolic turnover like synaptic

Discussion

compartments at 20% O_2. This assumption is supported by our data showing that redox responses as evoked in stratum radiatum are more sensitive to decreases in pO_2, which might imply an enhanced vulnerability of synaptic compartments during pathological processes in mitochondria.

5.5 Mitochondrial redox state during gamma oscillations

Changes in NAD(P)H fluorescence as evoked by gamma oscillations are characterized by long-lasting overshoots, although the interstitial pO_2 is clearly hyperoxic. This might represent an increase in substrate availability as a result of enhanced glycolysis in neuronal and astrocytic compartments (Kasischke et al., 2004; Brennan et al., 2006). This suggestion is strengthened by our finding that gamma oscillations are associated with a substantially increased O_2 consumption and thus an increased metabolic demand.

Other studies suggest that astrocytes provide lactate to neurons (Magistretti and Pellerin, 1999) by converting pyruvate into lactate during aerobic glycolysis and subsequently converting NADH into NAD^+. Based on the fact that interstitial pO_2 during gamma oscillations is in the normoxic range, neurons are supposed to use lactate as a preferred energy substrate even under aerobic conditions (Magistretti and Pellerin, 1999; Schurr et al., 1999). In line with this assumption, it has been suggested that astroglial gap junctions provide an activity-dependent intercellular pathway for the fast delivery of energy metabolites to neurons (Rouach et al., 2008).

The imbalance of neuronal TCA cycle and mitochondrial ETC activities and/or the partial inhibition of the ETC by free radicals (Brown, 2001; Erecinska and Silver, 2001) could be further explanations for the increase in NAD(P)H fluorescence as evoked by gamma oscillations.

In line with our finding that redox responses as evoked in stratum radiatum are more sensitive to decreases in pO_2, we have demonstrated that mitochondrial redox responses evoked by gamma oscillations are also larger in stratum radiatum. This probably reflects a higher metabolic demand in pre- and postsynaptic structures and perhaps increased enzyme activity and/or mitochondrial density (Wong-Riley, 1989; Waagepertersen et al., 1999; Attwell and Iadecola, 2002).

Discussion

NAD(P)H and FAD fluorescence transients during gamma oscillations are similar but not equal to those observed during the 20% O_2 condition. They have been characterized by attenuation of NAD(P)H dips and absence of FAD peaks. In line with the discussion of increased substrate availability during gamma oscillations, this could be explained by enhanced glycolysis and TCA cycle activities and an increase of mitochondrial Ca^{2+} concentration (Kann and Kovács, 2007), which would result in additional reduction of dinucleotide pools relative to oxidation. Highly increased ETC activity which does not allow a further increase in mitochondrial oxidation could be another possibility.

Since NAD(P)H and FAD fluorescence transients during gamma oscillations show similarities to those during low pO_2 (20% O_2) and to those observed *in vivo* under hypoxic conditions (LaManna et al., 1984), one can speculate that the alterations are due to low local O_2 availability which might leads to a limitation of the oxidative capacity of the ETC even under hyperoxic conditions. This suggests that transient local hypoxic conditions occur in microdomains with high amount of respiring mitochondria and/or clusters of mitochondria (Jones, 1986; Wong-Riley, 1989; Erecinska and Silver, 2001).

Further studies with improved technologies might clarify whether fast neuronal network oscillations are associated with transient local hypoxia in such microdomains. Nevertheless, based on our data we suggest that gamma oscillations are associated with utilization of mitochondrial oxidative capacity near limit.

5.6 Rotenone-induced alterations in mitochondrial redox state

We have demonstrated that rotenone has fast effects on the mitochondrial redox state shown by an immediate substantial increase in NAD(P)H fluorescence. Beyond that, we have shown that gamma oscillations in OHSCs are very sensitive to complex I inhibition. In contrast, it was shown that rotenone application (1 µM, 20 min, submerged conditions) in acute hippocampal slices had only minor effects on neuronal excitability as determined by transient increases in $[K^+]_o$ during electrical stimulation (Schuchmann et al., 2001). Rotenone might foremost interfere with energy and neurotransmitter metabolism of fast-spiking interneurons that contain high levels of CC (Gulyás et al., 2006) and are essential for rhythmic synchronisation of neuronal activity during gamma oscillations (Bartos et al., 2007; Fuchs et al., 2007). Thus, the effect of rotenone is closely related to our finding that gamma

Discussion

oscillations are highly sensitive to decreases in interstitial pO_2, while electrically evoked neuronal activities are more resistant. This suggests that local complex I inhibition by rotenone has similar effects compared to decreases in tissue pO_2. This is supported by the finding that rotenone mimics hypoxia in adrenomedullary chromaffin cells (Thompson et al., 2007). Moreover, our data support the assumption that gamma oscillations critically depend on mitochondrial oxidative energy metabolism.

To test the hypothesis whether rotenone mimics local hypoxia we compared NAD(P)H and FAD fluorescence transients in rotenone-treated OHSCs with those during low pO_2 (20% O_2). Therefore, we established an *in vitro* model where rotenone is applied in a nanomolar range for 5 *div* for local and subtle inhibition of the mitochondrial complex I. In other studies it was shown that rotenone treatment for one hour (100 nM) leads to neuronal cell death in OHSCs when quantified after a few days (Xu et al., 2003; Schuh et al., 2008). Our data have demonstrated that lower concentrations of rotenone (10 nM for 5 *div*) do not lead to enhanced neuronal cell death but to altered mitochondrial redox responses. NAD(P)H fluorescence transients do not differ from controls but FAD fluorescence transients show reduced peak components which likely indicate a limitation of mitochondrial oxidative capacity. Moreover, this supports our observation that NAD(P)H and FAD fluorescence signals are not necessarily coupled. However, redox responses during chronic rotenone treatment show different properties compared to redox responses during low pO_2 which suggests that acute decreases in pO_2 implicate other processes compared to prolonged inhibition of the ETC. Interestingly, redox responses during chronic rotenone treatment show similarities to redox responses during gamma oscillations since FAD peaks are also significantly reduced. This might indicate that gamma oscillations and chronic complex I inhibition in OHSCs elicit comparable limitations in oxidative metabolism. A possible reason for the reduction of the FAD peak component during chronic rotenone treatment might be that the complex II is permanently upregulated which might lead to utilization of oxidative capacity near limit. In this case, neuronal activation would not lead to further oxidation. Another explanation might be that complex I inhibition leads to ROS formation, which was reported by Fato et al., 2008. However, in other studies rotenone failed to enhance ROS generation (Adam-Vizi, 2005) and even inhibits ROS release due to reverse electron transfer (Liu et al., 2002). In contrast to the FAD peak component, the dip component of NAD(P)H fluorescence transients in rotenone-treated OHSCs is not reduced. This might indicate that rotenone specifically inhibits mitochondrial function, since FAD fluorescence is more specific for mitochondria compared to NAD(P)H fluorescence (Kunz and Kunz, 1985; Huang et al., 2002).

Discussion

The results show that chronic inhibition of complex I leads to altered mitochondrial redox responses but not to enhanced neuronal cell death suggesting a limitation of mitochondrial oxidative capacity.

Further experiments have to be performed to determine the metabolic demand in rotenone-treated OHSCs and to test whether it is possible to induce gamma oscillations in these slice cultures. The experiments will be helpful to refine this model to get a useful tool for studying local hypoxia in brain tissue.

5.7 Functional consequences

We have shown that gamma oscillations are associated with high O_2 consumption and that they are very sensitive to decreases in interstitial tissue pO_2. Therefore, we propose that even moderate decreases in pO_2 lead to significant disturbance of neuronal network activity which might explain the rapid loss of consciousness, an impaired ability to perform complex tasks and/or an impaired short-term memory (Verweij et al., 2007) and the occurrence of electroencephalographic slow-wave activity during brain ischemia, whereas evoked responses and ion distributions are more resistant (Hansen, 1985; Howard et al., 1998). We propose that fast neuronal network oscillations rely on outstanding functional performance of neuronal mitochondria (Buzsáki and Draguhn, 2004; Bartos et al., 2007). Mitochondrial dysfunction acts as a critical factor for the exceptional vulnerability of complex brain functions that might occur during aging, ischemia, neurodegenerative and psychiatric diseases (Erecinska and Silver, 2001; Pathak and Davey, 2008; Uhlhaas et al., 2008).

Our study highlights the importance of a functional understanding of mitochondria and their implications on activities on individual neurons and neuronal networks in health and disease.

6 Summary

Fast neuronal network oscillations in the gamma range (~30–80 Hz) have been implicated in higher brain functions such as memory formation, sensory processing and perhaps consciousness.

In hippocampal slice preparations, gamma oscillations can be evoked by ACh which mimics cholinergic input from the septum. In the hippocampal CA3 subfield, gamma oscillations arise from the precise interplay of action potential firing of excitatory glutamatergic principal neurons and fast inhibitory GABAergic interneurons. As a consequence, alternating pairs of current sinks and sources occur in stratum pyramidale and stratum radiatum, which require enhanced activation of Na^+/K^+-ATPases to restore ionic gradients and to maintain excitability. Thus, we hypothesized that gamma oscillations might critically depend on sufficient neuronal ATP supply.

In this study, the O_2 and energy demands of gamma oscillations were determined in acute mouse hippocampal slices and in rat OHSCs by applying electrophysiology, O_2 sensor microelectrodes and fluorescence imaging (NAD(P)H, FAD).

It was shown that persistent cholinergic gamma oscillations have similar properties in acute mouse hippocampal slices and in rat OHSCs. Further, it was demonstrated that gamma oscillations as well as spontaneous network activity decrease significantly at pO_2 levels that do not affect neuronal population responses as elicited by electrical stimuli. This leads to the suggestion that gamma oscillations are highly O_2 dependent. It is supported by our finding that gamma oscillations are associated with high levels of O_2 consumption. This is more prominent in area CA3 compared to CA1 and dentate gyrus. Moreover, gamma oscillations of high power require utilization of mitochondrial oxidative capacity near limit and are very sensitive to selective complex I inhibition by rotenone.

Furthermore, it was shown that chronic application of rotenone in the nanomolar range leads to alterations in mitochondrial redox responses that are not due to enhanced neuronal cell death, and that are similar to those evoked during gamma oscillations. This indicates that local and chronic inhibition of the ETC and persistent gamma oscillations elicit similar alterations in mitochondrial redox potentials. This leads to the assumption that both conditions might provoke limitations in oxidative capacity.

Summary

The data suggest that gamma oscillations are highly oxygen consuming and thus proper mitochondrial function is of major importance for fast neuronal network oscillations. We propose that mitochondrial dysfunction leads to disturbances of complex brain functions that might occur during aging, ischemia, neurodegenerative, and psychiatric diseases.

7 Zusammenfassung

Gamma-Oszillationen sind schnelle neuronale Netzwerkoszillationen im Bereich von ~30-80 Hz, die bei höheren Hirnfunktionen, wie Gedächtnisbildung und sensorischer Verarbeitung und eventuell während Prozessen, die bei der Bewusstseinsbildung auftreten, eine Rolle spielen.

In hippocampalen Schnittpräparaten können Gamma-Oszillationen mit Acetylcholin induziert werden. Dies spiegelt die cholinerge Projektion vom Septum zum Hippocampus *in vivo* wider. So entstehen in der CA3 Region Gamma-Oszillationen aus einem präzisen Zusammenspiel von Aktionspotentialen der exzitatorischen glutamatergen Pyramidenzellen und der schnellen inhibitorischen GABAergen Interneurone. Daraus folgt ein wechselseitiges An- und Absteigen der Ströme im Stratum Radiatum und Stratum Pyramidale. Dies erfordert eine erhöhte Aktivierung der Na^+/K^+-ATPase, um den Ionengradienten und somit die Erregbarkeit aufrecht zu erhalten. Daher liegt die Vermutung nahe, dass Gamma-Oszillationen im besonderen Maße auf neuronale ATP-Versorgung angewiesen sind.

In dieser Studie wurde der Sauerstoff- und Energiebedarf von Gamma-Oszillationen in akuten hippocampalen Schnittpräparaten von Mäusen und in organotypischen hippocampalen Schnittkulturen von Ratten mit elektrophysiologischen Methoden, sauerstoffsensitiven Elektroden und Fluoreszenzmessungen (NAD(P)H, FAD) untersucht.

Es konnte gezeigt werden, dass cholinerge Gamma-Oszillationen in den unterschiedlichen Schnittpräparaten ähnliche Eigenschaften besitzen. Ein weiterer Befund dieser Studie ist, dass ein reduzierter Sauerstoffpartialdruck keinen Effekt auf Feldpotentiale hat, die durch elektrische Stimulation induziert werden. Gamma-Oszillationen und spontane Netzwerkaktivität sind hingegen sehr stark von der umgebenden Sauerstoffkonzentration abhängig. Dies wird durch den Befund unterstützt, dass Gamma-Oszillationen einen sehr hohen Sauerstoffverbrauch haben. Während andauernder Oszillationen ist der Sauerstoffverbrauch in der CA3 Region am größten, in der CA1 Region und im Gyrus Dentatus ist er signifikant geringer.

Unsere Ergebnisse lassen vermuten, dass während anhaltender Gamma-Oszillationen die mitochondriale oxidative Kapazität ausgeschöpft ist. Darüber hinaus führt die Inhibition des Komplex I der Atmungskette mit Rotenon zu einer schnellen Reduzierung der Amplitude der Gamma-Oszillationen.

Zusammenfassung

Des Weiteren führt eine chronische Applikation von Rotenon im nanomolaren Bereich zu Veränderungen der mitochondrialen Redoxantworten, die jedoch nicht auf einen erhöhten neuronalen Zelltod zurückzuführen sind. Die Redoxantworten während chronischer Komplex I Inhibition und während anhaltender Gamma-Oszillationen haben ähnliche Eigenschaften. Dies zeigt, dass eine lokale und chronische Inhibition der Elektronentransportkette und anhaltende Gamma-Oszillationen vergleichbare Veränderungen des mitochondrialen Redoxpotentials auslösen und es deutet darauf hin, dass beide Situationen zu einer erheblichen Limitierung der oxidativen Kapazität führen können.

Die vorliegende Studie verdeutlicht, dass Gamma-Oszillationen einen hohen Sauerstoffverbrauch haben. Dies führt zu der Annahme, dass erhöhte mitochondriale Aktivität und/oder eine ausreichende Anzahl an Mitochondrien maßgeblich für anhaltende, schnelle Netzwerkoszillationen sind. Davon ausgehend, könnte eine Beeinträchtigung von mitochondrialen Funktionen zu Störungen von komplexen Hirnfunktionen führen, die möglicherweise im Alter, während einer Ischämie oder während neurodegenerativen und psychischen Krankheiten auftreten können.

8 References

Acker T and Acker H. Cellular oxygen sensing need in CNS function: physiological and pathological implications. J Experimental Biol. 2004; 207: 3171-3188.

Ackermann RF, Finch DM, Babb TL, Engel Jr J. Increased glucose metabolism during long-duration recurrent inhibition of hippocampal pyramidal cells. J Neurosci. 1984; 4: 251-264.

Adam-Vizi V. Production of reactive oxygen species in brain mitochondria: contribution by electron transport chain and non-electron transport chain sources. Antioxidants and Redox Signaling. 2005; 7(9+10): 1140-1149.

Aika Y, Ren JQ, Kosaka K, Kosaka T. Quantitative analysis of GABA-like-immunoreactive and parvalbumin-containing neurons in the CA1 region of the rat hippocampus using a stereological method, the dissector. Exp Brain Res. 1994; 99: 267-276.

Alam M and Schmidt WJ. Rotenone destroys dopaminergic neurons and induces parkinsonian symptoms in rats. Behav Brain Res. 2002; 136: 317-324.

Andersen P, Morris R, Amaral D, Bliss T, O'Keefe J. The Hippocampus Book. Oxford University Press. 2007; chapter 3, page 46.

Andrews ZB, Diano S, Horvath TL. Mitochondrial uncoupling proteins in the CNS: in support of function and survival. Nat Rev Neurosci. 2005; 6: 829-840.

Attwell D and Iadecola C. The neural basis of functional brain imaging signals. Trends Neurosci. 2002 Dec; 25(12): 621-625.

Aubin JE. Autofluorescence of viable cultured mammalian cells. J Histochem Cytochem. 1979; 27: 36-43.

Ayata C, Shin HK, Salomone S, Ozdemir-Gursoy Y, Boas DA, Dunn AK, Moskowitz MA. Pronounced hypoperfusion during spreading depression in mouse cortex. J Cereb Blood Flow Metab. 2004; 24: 1172-1182.

Bahr BA, Kessler M, Rivera S, Vanderklish PW, Hall RA, Mutneja MS, Gall C, Hoffmann KB. Stable maintenance of glutamate receptors and other synaptic components in long-term hippocampal slices. Hippocampus. 1995; 5: 425-439.

Bartos M, Vida I, Jonas P. Synaptic mechanisms of synchronized gamma oscillations in inhibitory interneuron networks. Nat Rev Neurosci. 2007 Jan; 8(1): 45-56.

Berger F, Ramirez-Hernandez MH, Ziegler M. The new life of a centenarian: signalling functions of NAD(P). Trends Biochem Sci. 2004; 29: 111-118.

References

Betarbet R, Sherer TB, MacKenzie G, Garcia-Osuna M, Panov AV, Greenamyre JT. Chronic systemic pesticide exposure reproduces features of Parkinson's disease. Nat Neurosci. 2000; 3(12): 1601-1306.

Both M, Bähner F, von Bohlen und Halbach O, Draguhn A. Propagation of specific network patterns through the mouse hippocampus. Hippocampus. 2008; 18: 899-908.

Bragin A, Jando G, Nadasdy Z, Hetke J, Wise K, Buzsaki G. Gamma (40-100 Hz) oscillation in the hippocampus of the behaving rat. J Neurosci. 1995 Jan; 15(1 Pt 1): 47-60.

Bragin A, Engel Jr. J, Wilson CL, Fried I, Buzsáki G. High-Frequency Oscillations in Human Brain. Hippocampus. 1999; 9: 137-142.

Brennan AM, Connor JA, Shuttleworth CW. NAD(P)H fluorescence transients after synaptic activity in brain slices: predominant role of mitochondrial function. J Cereb Blood Flow Metab. 2006; 26: 1389-1406.

Brown GC. Regulation of mitochondrial respiration by nitric oxide inhibition of cytochrome c oxidase. Biochim Biophys Acta. 2001; 1504: 46-57.

Buzsáki G and Chrobak JJ. Temporal structure in spatially organized neuronal ensembles: a role for interneuronal networks. Current Opinion in Neurobiology. 1995; 5: 504-510.

Buzsáki G and Draguhn A. Neuronal oscillations in cortical networks. Science. 2004; 304: 1926-1929.

Caeser M and Aertsen AD. Morphological organization of rat hippocampal slice cultures. J Comparative Neurology. 1991; 307: 87-106.

Chance B, Cohen P, Jöbsis F, Schoener B. Intracellular oxidation-reduction states *in vivo*. Science. 1962; 137: 499-508.

Chance B, Schoener B, Oshino R, Itshak F, Nakase Y. Oxidation-reduction ratio studies of mitochondria in freeze-trapped samples. J Biol Chem. 1979; 254(11): 4764-4771.

Cobb SR, Bulters DO, Suchak S, Riedel G, Morris RG, Davies CH. Activation of nicotinic acetylcholine receptors patterns network activity in the rodent hippocampus. J Physiol. 1999; 518: 131-140.

Cobb SR and Davies CH. Cholinergic modulation of hippocampal cells and circuits. J Physiol. 2005; 562.1: 81-88.

Csicsvari J, Jamieson B, Wise KD, Buzsáki G. Mechanisms of gamma oscillations in the hippocampus of the behaving rat. Neuron. 2003; 37: 311-322.

D'Ambrosio R, Gordon DS, Winn HR. Differential role of KIR channel and Na(+)/K(+)-pump in the regulation of extracellular K(+) in rat hippocampus. J Neurophysiol. 2002; 87(1): 87-102.

References

De Simoni A, Griesinger CB, Edwards FA. Development of rat CA1 neurones in acute versus organotypic slices: role of experience in synaptic morphology and activity. J Physiol. 2003; 550.1: 35-147.

Djuricic B, Berger R, Paschen W. Protein synthesis and energy metabolism in hippocampal slices during extended (24 hours) recovery following different periods of ischemia. Metabolic Brain Disease. 1994; 9(4): 377-389.

Dringen R. Metabolism and functions of glutathione in brain. Prog Neurobiol. 2000; 62: 649-671.

Duchen MR. Ca^{2+}-dependent changes in the mitochondrial energetics in single dissociated mouse sensory neurons. Biochem J. 1992; 283: 41-50.

Engel AK, Kreiter AK, König P, Singer W. Synchronization of oscillatory neuronal responses between striate and extrastriate visual cortical areas of the cat. Proc Natl Acad Sci USA. 1991; 88: 6048-6052.

Engel AK, Fries P, Singer W. Dynamic predictions: Oscillations and synchrony in top-down processing. Nature Rev. 2001; 2: 704-716.

Erecinska M and Silver IA. Tissue oxygen tension and brain sensitivity to hypoxia. Respiration Physiology. 2001; 128: 263-276.

Fato R, Bergamini C, Leoni S, Lenaz G. Mitochondrial production of reactive oxygen species: Role of complex I and quinine analogues. Bio Factors. 2008; 32: 31-39.

Fellous JM and Sejnowski TJ. Cholinergic induction of oscillations in the hippocampal slice in the slow (0.5-2 Hz), theta (5-12 Hz), and gamma (35-70 Hz) bands. Hippocampus. 2000; 10: 187-197.

Feng ZC, Roberts Jr EL, Sick TJ, Rosenthal M. Depth profile of local oxygen tension and blood flow in rat cerebral cortex, white matter and hippocampus. Brain Res. 1988; 445: 280-288.

Fisahn A, Pike FG, Buhl EH, Paulsen O. Cholinergic induction of network oscillations at 40 Hz in the hippocampus *in vitro*. Nature. 1998; 394: 186-189.

Fischer Y. The hippocampal intrinsic network oscillator. J Physiol. 2003; 554.1: 156-174.

Förster E, Zhao S, Frotscher M. Laminating the hippocampus. Nature Rev Neurosci. 2006; 7: 259-267.

Foster KA, Beaver CJ, Turner DA. Interaction between tissue oxygen tension and NADH imaging during synaptic stimulation and hypoxia in rat hippocampal slices. Neurosci. 2005; 132: 645-657.

Freeman WJ. Distribution in time and space of prepyriform electrical activity. J Neurophysiol. 1959; 22: 644-665.

References

Freeman WJ. Spatial properties of an EEG event in the olfactory bulb and cortex. Electroencephalogr Clin Neurophysiol. 1978; 44: 586-605.

Freund TF and Buzsáki G. Interneurons of the hippocampus. Hippocampus. 1996; 6: 347-470.

Friedman A, Behrens CJ, Heinemann U. Cholinergic dysfunction in temporal lobe epilepsy. Epilepsia. 2007; 48, Suppl. 5: 126-130.

Fuchs EC, Doheny H, Faulkner H, Caputi A, Traub RD, Bibbig A, Kopell N, Whittington MA, Monyer H. Genetically altered AMPA-type glutamate receptor kinetics in interneurons disrupt long-range synchrony of gamma oscillation. Proc Natl Acad Sci USA. 2001 Mar 13; 98(6): 3571-3576.

Fuchs EC, Zivkovic AR, Cunningham MO, Middleton S, Lebeau FE, Bannerman DM, Rozov A, Whittington MA, Traub RD, Rawlins JN, Monyer H. Recruitment of parvalbumin-positive interneurons determines hippocampal function and associated behavior. Neuron. 2007; 53: 591-604.

Fujimura N, Tanaka E, Yamamoto S, Shigemori M, Higashi H. Contribution of ATP-sensitive potassium channels to hypoxic hyperpolarization in rat hippocampal CA1 neurons *in vitro*. J Neurophysiol. 1997; 77: 378-385.

Gaedicke R and Albus K. Real-time separation of multineuron recordings with a DSP32C signal processor. J Neurosci Methods. 1995; 57: 187-193.

Gerich FJ, Hepp S, Probst I, Müller M. Mitochondrial inhibition prior to oxygen-withdrawal facilitates the occurrence of hypoxia-induced spreading depression in rat hippocampal slices. J Neurophysiol. 2006; 96: 492-504.

Gjedde A. Cerebral blood flow change arterial hypoxemia is consistent with negligible oxygen tension in brain mitochondria. NeuroImage. 2002; 17: 1876-1881.

Gjedde A, Marrett S, Vafaee M. Oxidative and Nonoxidative Metabolism of Excited Neurons and Astrocytes. J Cerebral Blood Flow and Metabolism. 2002; 22: 1-14.

Gloveli T, Dugladze T, Saha S, Monyer H, Heinemann U, Traub RD, Whittington MA, Buhl EH. Differential involvement of oriens/pyramidale interneurones in hippocampal network oscillations in vitro. J Physiol. 2005; 562.1: 131-147.

Gray CM. Synchronous oscillations in neuronal systems: mechanisms and functions. J Comput Neurosci. 1994; 1: 11-38.

Gulyás AI, Buzsáki G, Freund TF, Hirase H. Populations of hippocampal inhibitory neurons express different levels of cytochrome c. Eur J Neurosci. 2006 May; 23(10): 2581-2594.

Gunter TE, Yule DI, Gunter KK, Eliseev RA, Salter JD. Calcium and mitochondria. FEBS Lett. 2004; 567: 96-102.

References

Gutierrez R and Heinemann U. Synaptic reorganization in explanted cultures of rat hippocampus. Brain Res. 1999; 815: 304-316.

Hájos N, Pálhalmi J, Mann EO, Németh B, Paulsen O, Freund TF. Spike timing of distinct types of GABAergic interneuron during hippocampal gamma oscillations *in vitro*. J Neurosci. 2004; 24(41): 9127-9137.

Hájos N, Ellender TJ, Zemankovics R, Mann EO, Exley R, Cragg SJ, Freund TF, Paulsen O. Spike timing of distinct types of GABAergic interneuron maintaining network activity in submerged hippocampal slices: importance of oxygen supply. Europ J Neurosci. 2009; 29: 319-327.

Hamon B, Stanton PK, Heinemann U. An N-methyl-D-aspartate receptor-independent excitatory action of partial reduction of extracellular [Mg^{2+}] in CA1-region of rat hippocampal slices. Neurosci Letters. 1987; 75: 240-245.

Hansen AJ. Effect of anoxia on ion distribution in the brain. Physiol Rev. 1985; 65: 101-148.

Hansford RG and Zorov D. Role of mitochondrial calcium transport in the control of substrate oxidation. Mol Cell Biochem. 1998; 184: 359-369.

Hayakawa Y, Nemoto T, Iino M, Kasai H. Rapid Ca^{2+} -dependent increase in oxygen consumption by mitochondria in single mammalian central neurons. Cell Calcium. 2005; 37: 359-370.

Heinemann U, Schaible HG, Schmidt RF. Changes in extracellular potassium concentration in cat spinal cord in response to innocuous and noxious stimulation of legs with healthy and inflamed knee joints. Exp Brain Res. 1990; 79(2): 283-292.

Heinemann U and Arens J. Production and calibration of ion-sensitive microelectrodes. In: Practical Electrophysiological Methods (Kettenmann H, Grantyn R, eds), Wiley-Liss, New York, USA. 1992; 206-212.

Heinemann U, Schmitz D, Eder C, Gloveli T. Properties of entorhinal cortex projection cells to the hippocampal formation. Ann N Y Acad Sci. 2000; 911: 112-126.

Hoffmann U, Pomper J, Graulich J, Zeller M, Schuchmann S, Gabriel S, Maier RF, Heinemann U. Changes of neuronal activity in areas CA1 and CA3 during anoxia and normoxic or hyperoxic reoxygenation in juvenile rat organotypic hippocampal slice cultures. Brain Res. 2006 Jan 19; 1069(1): 207-215. Epub 2005 Dec 27.

Holopainen IE. Organotypic Hippocampal Slice Cultures: A model system to study basic cellular and molecular mechanisms of neuronal cell death, neuroprotection, and synaptic plasticity. Neurochem Res. 2005; 30 (12): 1521-1528.

Howard EM, Gao TM, Pulsinelli WA, Xu ZC. Electrophysiological changes of CA3 neurons and dentate granule cells following transient forebrain ischemia. Brain Res. 1998; 798: 109-118.

References

Huang S, Heikal AA, Webb WW. Two-photon fluorescence spectroscopy and microscopy of NAD(P)H and flavoprotein. Biophys J. 2002; 82: 2811-2812.

Huchzermeyer C, Albus K, Gabriel HJ, Otáhal J, Taubenberger N, Heinemann U, Kovács R, Kann O. Gamma oscillations and spontaneous network activity in the hippocampus are highly sensitive to decreases in pO2 and concomitant changes in mitochondrial redox state. J Neurosci. 2008; 28(5): 1153-1162.

Jöbsis FF, O'Connor M, Vitale A, Vreman H. Intracellular redox changes in functioning cerebral cortex. I. Metabolic effects of epileptiform activity. J Neurophysiol. 1971; 34: 735-749.

Joliot M, Ribary U, Llinás R. Human oscillatory brain activity near 40 Hz coexists with cognitive temporal binding. Proc Natl Acad Sci USA. 1994; 91: 11748-11751.

Jones DP. Intracellular diffusion gradients of O2 and ATP. Am. J Physiol. 1986; 250 (19): C663-C675.

Kadenbach B. Intrinsic and extrinsic uncoupling of oxidative phosphorylation. Biochim Biophys Acta. 2003; 1604: 77-94.

Kann O, Schuchmann S, Buchheim K, Heinemann U. Coupling of neuronal activity and mitochondrial metabolism as revealed by NAD(P)H fluorescence signals in organotypic hippocampal slice cultures of the rat. Neurosci. 2003a; 119: 87-100.

Kann O, Kovács R, Heinemann U. Metabotropic receptor-mediated Ca^{2+} signaling elevates mitochondrial Ca^{2+} and stimulates oxidative metabolism in hippocampal slice cultures. J Neurophysiol. 2003b Aug; 90(2): 613-621.

Kann O, Kovács R, Njunting M, Behrens CJ, Otáhal J, Lehmann TN, Gabriel S, Heinemann. Metabolic dysfunction during neuronal activation in the ex vivo hippocampus from chronic epileptic rats and humans. Brain. 2005; 128: 2396-2407.

Kann O and Kovács R. Mitochondria and neuronal activity. Am J Physiol Cell Physiol. 2007 Feb; 292(2): C641-C657.
Kaplan NO. The role of pyridine nucleotides in regulating cellular metabolism. Curr Top Cell Regul. 1985; 26: 371-381.

Kasischke KA, Vishwasrao HD, Fisher PJ, Zipfel WR, Webb WW. Neural activity triggers neuronal oxidative metabolism followed by astrocytic glycolysis. Science. 2004; 305: 99-103.

Kirsch M and de Groot H. NAD(P)H, a directly operating antioxidant? FASEB J. 2001; 15: 1569-1574.

Klaidman LK, Mukherjee SK, Adams JD Jr. Oxidative changes in brain pyridine nucleotides and neuroprotection using nicotinamide. Biochim Biophys Acta. 2001; 1525: 136-148.

References

Klausberger T, Magill PJ, Marton LF, Roberts JD, Cobden PM, Buzsáki G, Somogyi P. Brain-state- and cell-type-specific firing of hippocampal interneurons *in vivo*. Nature. 2003; 421: 844-848.

Kovács R, Schuchmann S, Gabriel S, Kardos J, Heinemann U. Ca^{2+} signalling and changes of mitochondrial function during low-Mg^{2+}-induced epileptiform activity in organotypic hippocampal slice cultures. European J Neurosci. 2001; 13: 1311-1319.

Kovács R, Kardos J, Heinemann U, Kann O. Mitochondrial calcium ion and membrane potential transients follow the pattern of epileptiform discharges in hippocampal slice cultures. J Neurosci. 2005 Apr 27; 25(17): 4260-4269.

Kunz WS and Kunz W. Contribution of different enzymes to flavoprotein fluorescence of isolated rat liver mitochondria. Biochim Biophys Acta. 1985; 841: 237-246.

Kwong KK, Belliveau JW, Chesler DA, Goldberg IE, Weisskoff RM, Poncelet BP, Kennedy DN, Hoppel BE, Cohen MS, Turner R. Dynamic magnetic resonance imaging of human brain activity during primary sensory stimulation. Proc Natl Acad Sci USA. 1992; 89: 5675-5679.

LaManna JC, Light AI, Peretsman SJ, Rosenthal M. Oxygen insufficiency during hypoxic hypoxia in rat brain cortex. Brain Res. 1984; 293: 313-318.

LeBeau FE, Towers SK, Traub RD, Whittington MA, Buhl EH. Fast network oscillations induced by potassium transients in the rat hippocampus *in vitro*. J Physiol. 2002; 542(Pt 1): 167-179.

Lipinski HG. Model calculations of oxygen supply to tissue slice preparations. Phys Med Biol. 1989; 34(8): 1103-1111.

Lipton P. Effects on membrane depolarization on nicotinamide nucleotide fluorescence in brain slices. Biochem J. 1973; 136: 999-1009.

Liu Y, Fiskum G, Schubert D. Generation of reactive oxygen species by the mitochondrial electron transport chain. J Neurochem. 2002; 80: 780-787.

Lopes da Silva FH, Witter MP, Boeijinga PH, Lohman AHM. Anatomic organization and physiology of the limbic cortex. Physiol Rev. 1990; 70(2): 458-511.

MacDonald KD, Brett B, Barth DS. Inter- and intra-hemispheric spatiotemporal organization of spontaneous electrocortical oscillations. J Neurophysiol. 1996; 76: 423-437.

Magistretti PJ and Pellerin L. Cellular mechanisms of brain energy metabolism and their relevance to functional brain imaging. Phil Trans R Soc Lond B. 1999; 354: 1155-1163.

Mann EO, Suckling JM, Hajos N, Greenfield SA, Paulsen O. Perisomatic feedback inhibition underlies cholinergically induced fast network oscillations in the rat hippocampus *in vitro*. Neuron. 2005; 45: 105-117.

References

Mayevsky A and Chance B. Metabolic responses of the awake cerebral cortex to anoxia hypoxia spreading depression and epileptiform activity. Brain Res. 1975; 98: 149-165.

Mayevsky A and Chance B. Oxidation-reduction states of NADH *in vivo*: from animals to clinical use. Mitochondrion. 2007; 7: 330-339.

McCormack JG, Halestrap AP, Denton RM. Role of calcium ions in regulation of mammalian intramitochondrial metabolism. Physiol Rev. 1990; 70: 391-425.

Mironov SL and Richter DW. Oscillations and hypoxic changes of mitochondrial variables in neurons of the brainstem respiratory centre of mice. J Physiol. 2001; 533: 227-236.

Mody I, Lambert JDC, Heinemann U. Low extracellular magnesium induces epileptiform activity and spreading depression in rat hippocampal slices. J Neurophysiol. 1987; 57(3): 869-888.

Moroni F, Malthe-Sorenssen D, Cheney DL, Costa E. Modulation of ACh turnover in the septal-hippocampal pathway by electrical stimulation and lesioning. Brain Res. 1978; 150: 333-341.

Muravchick S and Levy RJ. Clinical implications of mitochondrial dysfunction. Anesthesiology. 2006; 105: 819-837.

Ndubuizu O and LaManna JC. Brain tissue oxygen concentration measurements. Antioxidants and Redox Signaling. 2007; 9(8): 1207-1219.

Newman EA, Frambach DA, Odette LL. Control of extracellular potassium levels by retinal glial cell K^+ siphoning. Science. 1984; 225(4667): 1174-1175.

Niessing J, Ebisch B, Schmidt KE, Niessing M, Singer W, Galuske RA. Hemodynamic signals correlate tightly with synchronized gamma oscillations. Science. 2005; 309: 948-951.
Offenhauser N, Thomsen K, Caesar K, Lauritzen M. Activity-induced tissue oxygenation changes in rat cerebellar cortex: interplay of postsynaptic activation and blood flow.
J Physiol (Lond). 2005; 565: 279-294.

Ogawa S, Lee TM, Kay AR, Tank DW. Brain magnetic resonance imaging with contrast dependent on blood oxygenation. Proc Natl Acad Sci USA. 1990; 87: 9868-9872.

Ogawa S, Tank DW, Menon R, Ellermann JM, Kim SG, Merkle H, Ugurbil K. Intrinsic signal changes accompanying sensory stimulation: functional brain mapping with magnetic resonance imaging. Proc Natl Acad Sci USA. 1992; 89: 5951-5955.

O'Keefe J. A review of the hippocampal place cells. Progress in Neurobiology. 1979; 13: 419-439.

Pálhalmi J, Paulsen O, Freund TF, Hájos N. Distinct properties of carbachol- and DHPG-induced network oscillations in hippocampal slices. Neuropharmacology. 2004; 47: 381-389.

References

Pathak RU and Davey GP. complex I and energy thresholds in the brain. Biochim Biophys Acta. 2008 Jul-Aug; 1777(7-8): 777-782.

Pomper JK, Haack S, Petzold GC, Buchheim K, Gabriel S, Hoffmann U, Heinemann U. Repetitive spreading depression-like events result in cell damage in juvenile hippocampal slice cultures maintained in normoxia. J Neurophysiol. 2006; 95: 355-368.

Popov V, Medvedev NI, Davies HA, Stewart MG. Mitochondria form a filamentous reticular network in hippocampal dendrites but are present as discrete bodies in axons: a three-dimensional ultrastructural study. J Comp Neurol. 2005; 492: 50-65.

Ribary U, Ioannides AA, Singh KD, Hasson R, Bolton JP, Laado F, Mogilner A, Llinás R. Magnetic field tomography of coherent thalamocortical 40 Hz oscillations in humans. Proc Natl Acad Sci USA. 1994; 88: 11037-11041.

Rolett EL, Azzawi A, Liu KJ, Yongbi MN, Swartz HM, Dunn JF. Critical oxygen tension in rat brain: a combined (31)P-NMR and EPR oximetry study. Am J Physiol Regul integr Comp Physiol. 2000; 279: R9-R16.

Rolfe DFS and Brown GC. Cellular energy utilization and molecular origin of standard metabolic rate in mammals. Physiol Rev. 1997; 77: 731-758.

Rouache N, Koulakoff A, Abudara V, Willecke K, Giaume C. Astroglial metabolic networks sustain hippocampal synaptic transmission. Science. 2008; 322: 1551-1555.

Scholz R, Thurman RG, Williamson JR, Chance B, Bucher T. Flavin and pyridine nucleotide oxidation-reduction changes in perfused rat liver. J Biol Chem. 1969; 244: 2317-2324.

Schuchmann S, Kovács R, Kann O, Heinemann U, Buchheim K. Monitoring NAD(P)H autofluorescence to assess mitochondrial metabolic functions in rat hippocampal-entorhinal cortex slices. Brain Res Protoc. 2001; 7: 267-276.

Schmued LC and Hopkins KJ. Fluoro-Jade B: a high affinity fluorescent marker for the localization of neuronal degeneration. Brain Res. 2000; 874: 123-130.

Schuh RA, Matthews CC, Fishman PS. Interaction of mitochondrial respiratory inhibitors and excitotoxins potentiates cell death in hippocampal slice cultures. J Neurosci Res. 2008; 86: 3306-3313.

Schurr A, Miller JJ, Payne RS, Rigor BM. An increase in lactate output by brain tissue serves to meet the energy needs of glutamate-activated neurons. J Neurosci. 1999; 19(1): 34-39.

Shuttleworth CW, Brennan AM, Connor JA. NAD(P)H fluorescence imaging of postsynaptic neuronal activation in murine hippocampal slices. J Neurosci. 2003; 23: 3196-3208.

Singer W. Synchronization of cortical activity and its putative role in information processing and learning. Annu Rev Physiol. 1993; 55: 349-374.

References

Stenkamp K, Palva JM, Uusisaari M, Schuchmann S, Schmitz D, Heinemann U, Kaila K. Enhanced temporal stability of cholinergic hippocampal gamma oscillations following respiratory alkalosis in vitro. J Neurophysiol. 2001; 85: 2063-2069.

Stewart M and Fox SE. Do septal neurons pace the hippocampal theta rhythm? Trends Neurosci. 1990; 13: 163-168.

Stoppini L, Buchs PA, Muller D. A simple method for organotypic cultures of nervous tissue. J Neurosci Methods. 1991 Apr; 37(2): 173-182.

Takano T, Tian GF, Peng W, Lou N, Lovatt D, Hansen AJ, Kasischke KA, Nedergaard M. Cortical spreading depression causes and coincides with tissue hypoxia. Nat Neurosci; 2007; 10: 754-762.

Tata DA and Anderson BJ. A new method for the investigation of capillary structure. J Neurosci Methods. 2002; 113: 199-206.

Thompson JK, Peterson MR, Freeman RD. Single-neuron activity and tissue oxygenation in the cerebral cortex. Science. 2003; 299: 1070-1072.

Thompson RJ, Buttigieg J, Zhang M, Nurse CA. A rotenone-sensitive site and H_2O_2 are key components of hypoxia-sensing in neonatal rat adrenomedullary chromaffin cells. Neurosci. 2007; 145: 130-141.

Tukker JJ, Fuentealba P, Hartwich K, Somogyi P, Klausberger T. Cell type-specific tuning of hippocampal interneuron firing during gamma oscillations *in vivo*. J Neurosci. 2007; 27(31): 8184-8189.

Turner DA, Foster KA, Galeffi F, Somjen GG. Differences in O_2 availability resolve the apparent discrepencies in metabolic intrinsic optical signals *in vivo* and *in vitro*. Trends Neurosci. 2007; 30: 390-398.

Uhlhaas PJ, Haenschel C, Nikolić D, Singer W. The role of oscillations and synchrony in cortical networks and their putative relevance for the pathophysiology of schizophrenia. Schizophr Bull. 2008 Sep; 34(5): 927-943.

Verstreken P, Ly CV, Venken KJ, Koh TW, Zhou Y, Bellen HJ. Synaptic mitochondria are critical for mobilization of reverse pool vesicles at *Drosophila* neuromuscular junctions. Neuron. 2005; 47: 365-378.

Verweij BH, Amelink GJ, Muizelaar JP. Current concepts of cerebral oxygen transport and energy metabolism after severe traumatic brain injury. Progress in Brain Res. 2007; 161: 111-124.

Wang T and Kass IS. Preparation of brain slices. Methods Mol Biol. 1997; 72: 1-14.

Waagepetersen HS, Sonnewald U, Schousboe A. The GABA paradox: multiple roles as metabolite, neurotransmitter, and neurodifferentiative agent. J Neurochem. 1999; 73: 1335-1342.

References

Whittington MA, Stanford IM, Colling SB, Jefferys JG, Traub RD. Spatiotemporal patterns of gamma frequency oscillations tetanically induced in the rat hippocampal slice. J Physiol. 1997 Aug 1; 502 (Pt 3): 591-607.

Whittington MA, Faulkner HJ, Doheny HC, Traub RD. Neuronal fast oscillations as a target site for psychoactive drugs. Pharmacology and Therapeutics. 2000; 86: 171-190.

Williams JH and Kauer JA. Properties of carbachol-induced oscillatory activity in rat hippocampus. J Neurophysiol. 1997; 78: 2631-2640.

Witter MP and Amaral DG. Hippocampal Formation. The Rat Nervous System, Third Edition, 2004; Chapter 21.

Wójtowicz AM, van den Boom L, Chakrabarty A, Maggio N, ul Haq R, Behrens CJ, Heinemann U. Monoamines block kainate- and carbachol-induced gamma oscillations but augment stimulus-induced gamma oscillations in rat hippocampus *in vitro*. Hippocampus. 2009; 19: 273-288.

Wong-Riley MT. Cytochrome oxidase: an endogenous metabolic marker for neuronal activity. Trends Neurosci. 1989 Mar; 12(3): 94-101.

Woodson W, Nitecka L, Ben-Ari Y. Organization of the GABAergic system in the rat hippocampa formation: a quantitative immunocytochemical study. J Comp Neurol. 1989; 280: 254-271.

Xu G, Perez-Pinzon MA, Sick TJ. Mitochondrial complex I inhibition produces selective damage to hippocampal subfield CA1 in organotypic slice cultures. Neurotoxicity Res. 2003; 5(7): 529-538.

Yamada K, Ji JJ, Yuan H, Miki T, Sato S, Horimoto N, Shimizu T, Seino S, Inagaki N. Protective role of ATP-sensitive potassium channels in hypoxia-induced generalized seizure. Science. 2001; 292: 1543-1546.

Zauner A, Daugherty WP, Bullock MR, Warner DS. Brain oxygenation and energy metabolism: Part I-Biological function and pathophysiology. Neurosurgery. 2002; 51: 289-302.

9 Acknowledgments

Foremost, I like to thank Prof. Uwe Heinemann for supervising my PhD thesis, for scientific support, and for giving me the opportunity to work in his lab.

I am very thankful to PD Dr. Oliver Kann for excellent mentoring and valuable advice in the matter of organizing lab work and scientific writing.

Special thanks to Dr. Richard Kovács for helping building up the setups, for valuable criticism to this thesis and for motivating scientific discussions.

I am particularly grateful to Kristin Lehmann for exceptional technical assistance.

I am pleased to thank Dr. Hans-Jürgen Gabriel for helping me with the oxygen measurements.

I gratefully acknowledge my collaborators Prof. Markus Schuelke, Stefanie Wirtz and Anja Brinckmann from the Department of Neuropediatrics.

Many colleagues contributed to this work by helping me with the experiments, sharing lab equipment, helping with computer problems and organization. Special thanks to: Prof. Klaus Albus, Nando Taubenberger, Dr. Jakub Otáhal, Dr. Herbert Siegmund, Agustin Liotta, Ibrahim Zarour, Dr. Katrin Schulze, Sonja Frosinski, Andrea Schütz and Bernd Schacht.

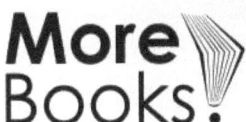
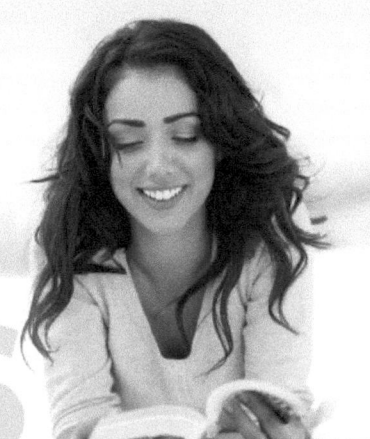

I want morebooks!

Buy your books fast and straightforward online - at one of world's fastest growing online book stores! Environmentally sound due to Print-on-Demand technologies.

Buy your books online at
www.morebooks.shop

Kaufen Sie Ihre Bücher schnell und unkompliziert online – auf einer der am schnellsten wachsenden Buchhandelsplattformen weltweit! Dank Print-On-Demand umwelt- und ressourcenschonend produziert.

Bücher schneller online kaufen
www.morebooks.shop

KS OmniScriptum Publishing
Brivibas gatve 197
LV-1039 Riga, Latvia
Telefax: +371 686 204 55

info@omniscriptum.com
www.omniscriptum.com

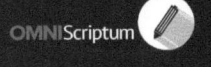

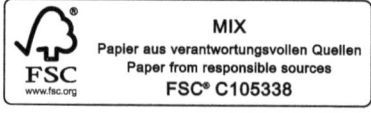

Printed by Books on Demand GmbH, Norderstedt / Germany